The Insider's Pocket Guide to Navigating a Faculty Career in Academic Medicine

Heather Brod • Kimberly Skarupski

The Insider's Pocket Guide to Navigating a Faculty Career in Academic Medicine

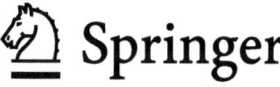

Heather Brod
Heather Brod LLC, Columbus, OH, USA

Kimberly Skarupski
Office of Faculty Affairs
University of Texas Medical Branch
Galveston, TX, USA

ISBN 978-3-031-66098-6   ISBN 978-3-031-66096-2 (eBook)
https://doi.org/10.1007/978-3-031-66096-2

© The Editor(s) (if applicable) and The Author(s), under exclusive license to Springer Nature Switzerland AG 2024

This work is subject to copyright. All rights are solely and exclusively licensed by the Publisher, whether the whole or part of the material is concerned, specifically the rights of translation, reprinting, reuse of illustrations, recitation, broadcasting, reproduction on microfilms or in any other physical way, and transmission or information storage and retrieval, electronic adaptation, computer software, or by similar or dissimilar methodology now known or hereafter developed.

The use of general descriptive names, registered names, trademarks, service marks, etc. in this publication does not imply, even in the absence of a specific statement, that such names are exempt from the relevant protective laws and regulations and therefore free for general use.

The publisher, the authors and the editors are safe to assume that the advice and information in this book are believed to be true and accurate at the date of publication. Neither the publisher nor the authors or the editors give a warranty, expressed or implied, with respect to the material contained herein or for any errors or omissions that may have been made. The publisher remains neutral with regard to jurisdictional claims in published maps and institutional affiliations.

This Springer imprint is published by the registered company Springer Nature Switzerland AG
The registered company address is: Gewerbestrasse 11, 6330 Cham, Switzerland

If disposing of this product, please recycle the paper.

This book is dedicated to all the faculty members in academic medicine—those before us, with us now, and those who will come after us—who have dedicated their life's work in service to education, mentorship, discovery, prevention, diagnosis, treatment, and cures. We are grateful to all those who have shared their stories so that others may learn. The contributions made by faculty at academic medical centers are noble, bold, courageous, and life-saving. To the extent that we can ease, in even a small way, the enormous pressure that our faculty face each day is an endeavor worth undertaking.

Introduction

It is 3 pm on a Friday afternoon and I (Heather)[1] am meeting with an early-career faculty member about her desire to do more teaching in her department. She tells me that when she was interviewed 2 years ago, teaching was discussed and she doesn't understand why the department keeps putting her off. I looked her up prior to our meeting and saw that she is on a track that is strictly clinical, so I am confused as to why she would think that a more significant teaching load is forthcoming. However, one never knows, so I ask what her letter of offer says. "Letter of offer?" Her puzzlement increases, "I don't know, that was just something I signed."

I clarify that a letter of offer documents her faculty track, assigns workload, and comprises a baseline set of expectations and the agreed-upon promises. I further describe that there are several different faculty tracks, and each one has a different set of expectations. By her title, it appears that she's on a track that is used for people who exclusively provide clinical service.

All of this is news to her. I am unfortunately not surprised. Many faculty members accept positions in academic medicine with very little awareness of the world of academic medicine. Throughout our combined nearly six decades of experience in academia, we have met thousands of faculty members at different points in their careers, from pre-hire to retirement. Often, faculty members schedule meetings with us when they find themselves wanting or expecting something other than their current reality and not knowing how to go about getting it. Like detectives, we are professional dot-connectors, identifying root causes of disconnect, the impetus behind goals, and the best approaches for matching a faculty members' professional growth and achievement to an organization's needs and expectations.

A couple weeks after our first meeting, the early-career faculty member who wanted to teach more was in my office again. She had her letter of offer. "You're right," she said, "this says that I'm clinical and that I *may* be considered for teaching opportunities as they arise." She looked crestfallen. Her expectation, the reason she

---

[1] As this book is a co-authorship, we will use "we" when referring to our combined or shared experiences and an undifferentiated "I" when describing individual experiences.

accepted the role, was that she wanted to teach. It is not an unreasonable expectation to think that working at an academic medical center would yield teaching opportunities, so she had not bothered to read the fine print and likely was so excited about the promise of teaching that she had not heard the qualifiers.

She wanted to know whether there was anything she could do to get some teaching opportunities. As her clinical career track was a limitation to teaching opportunities at the college level, we discussed how she could approach the chairperson of her department about changing tracks. I was unaware of what her departmental constraints might be and so we strategized her pitch, namely to be mindful of budget and release time, identifying who else could take on responsibilities she currently held, and to focus on the educational gaps her expertise fulfilled and what benefits the department could receive from filling them.

A week later, she called. It was a no-go. The chair had told her that she had accepted the job as described in the offer letter offered and that she was needed in that clinical role. She was devastated. However, a carrot had been dangled—should a position with teaching responsibilities open up, she would be considered for it. Over the next several months, the early-career faculty member tried to remain optimistic, engaged in all the volunteer teaching she could, and became increasingly resentful about doing uncompensated work and feeling brushed-aside by the chair. After about a year, she called again, this time to say that she was leaving the institution for a position at another academic medical center that came with teaching responsibilities.

Unfortunately, we have seen too many academic careers cut short, mismanaged, or stalled due to a lack of alignment between the faculty member and the organization's expectations. Feeling like your expertise and potential are being squandered is a surefire path to frustration and burnout, which often results in job-hopping or exiting academia altogether. We invest too much of our valuable time, effort, and resources training to become physicians, scientists, psychologists, epidemiologists, physical therapists, educators, and the many other types of health care professionals for our careers to flounder or fail.

Fortunately, our early-career faculty member was not disillusioned by academic medicine entirely; she learned some hard lessons but found a dream position at another university. Nevertheless, one might wonder how a win–win solution may have been achieved—and that is why we wanted to write this book—to help others from having to learn these lessons the hard way.

The good news is that it does not need to be so hard. As faculty affairs and development professionals, we have spent a significant portion of our careers creating comprehensive career development strategies and tactics. We have mediated conflicts, provided mentorship, sponsorship and coaching, given advice, developed and presented innumerable workshops, revised dossiers, taught leadership skills, talked faculty members off proverbial ledges, brokered deals, repaired bruised egos, and emphasized, time and time again, the importance of impact.

And it must be pointed out that we have not done this alone. Through engagement with the Association of American Medical Colleges (AAMC) Group on Faculty Affairs and via Kim's *Faculty Factory* podcast, we both have sat at many tables with our faculty affairs and faculty development colleagues from the 171 accredited U.S. and Canadian medical schools [1] wrestling with the myriad challenges of helping faculty create thriving careers that enrich the institutions we collectively serve. It is with great gratitude to these colleagues that we present this book, knowing that our thinking and expertise have been shaped by their knowledge and generosity in sharing their experiences such that we may all learn.

One of the constant struggles for faculty affairs and faculty development professionals is cutting through the noise. We are the big picture people; our work asks faculty members to consider the "important, but not urgent" quadrant of the Eisenhower matrix (Stephen Covey, in his famous book, *The 7 Habits of Highly Effective People,* used Dwight D. Eisenhower's words to create the now famous time management matrix). The "important, but not urgent" quadrant is the quadrant of quality and personal leadership. It's the space where potential is realized and jobs flourish into careers. However, there is so much pressure with dashboards and metrics, grant application deadlines, manuscripts in progress, teaching and mentoring obligations, programs to develop, service projects, and countless administrative responsibilities that faculty members rarely dedicate focused time to this leadership quadrant. In effect, contemporary faculty members juggle the responsibilities equivalent to holding four jobs in one—not counting home life, which may include child and/or parental care. The academic medicine work culture is unique in how it sets extraordinarily high expectation bars coupled with a low-no resource ecosystem. This environment unfortunately results in a state of constant busyness which oftentimes leads faculty members to lose sight of the big picture, because there's always something "urgent" (though not always "important") vying for their attention. Therefore, we aimed to create this resource for you that is simple, relatively brief, widely available, scalable, asynchronous, and tailored to meet you exactly where you are.

The result is this book that focuses on faculty members' needs and experiences. The topics presented here are the subjects that we are most often asked to meet about, present on, and develop into workshops. We have presented the topics here in a format designed to bridge the knowing-doing gap. If there is one takeaway message of this entire book, it is that focusing attention on the important—and oftentimes neglected—career and professional development work is what yields fulfilling, aligned, and successful careers.

This book is intended as an aid for any type of career exploration from new hire out of fellowship or post-doc through mid- or late-career transitions. Importantly, we feature stories and examples from your colleagues in all types of roles across the tripartite missions of education, research, and health care. We also provide supplemental worksheets and links to additional resources on Heather's website: www.heatherbrod.com. In Chap. 1, we provide a systematic overview of academic medicine, with a focus on the "why." Chapter 2 describes how to train for an academic medicine career and then how to translate the training and your interests toward applying for specific roles. In our field, it is often said that if you know one academic medical center, you know one academic medical center. Each institution has its own nuances, and yet, there are some common systemic and institutional factors that can be illuminated by informed inquiry and effective decision-making.

In Chap. 3, we encourage you to explore who you are, which is distinct from what you do! We walk you through the development of vision and mission statements that incorporate your values, strengths, and utilize essential skills like emotional intelligence. Chapter 4 provides insights into how you can get the right position for you by doing some old-fashioned research to determine both *what* you want to do and *where* you should do it. We share job search strategies and an overview of the common academic faculty tracks, along with negotiating job offers. Chapter 5 talks about onboarding—for first-time faculty, for being new to an institution, and for being new to any role. We describe how networking is an important strategy for acclimating to a new culture, how to find mentors and be a good mentee, developing organizational savvy, and preparing for promotion.

Chapter 6 addresses the fundamental "academic" component of academic medicine, namely science and scholarship. We present tools like writing accountability groups (WAGs) and time management strategies to help you develop sustainable scholarly habits. Chapter 7 is dedicated to promotion—the policies, criteria, and processes. We also address leadership opportunities and general career advancement as faculty members advance through the promotional ranks. In Chap. 8, we discuss leadership and what constitutes good leadership. We point you to leadership competencies, programs, and content. Chapter 9 addresses the inevitable hurdles and challenges in academic medicine. We discuss common scenarios including professional misconduct, mid-career malaise, burnout, setbacks, and help you identify the warning signs for "rough road ahead." We also point to coaching as a strategy to overcome obstacles. Chapter 10 illuminates how employing a diversity- and inclusive-mindset enhances our well-being, productivity, and careers. In Chap. 11, we present the work–life integration paradox and discuss strategies that will help you enjoy both work life and home life. Finally, in Chap. 12, we present career and life transition points and discuss how gains and losses will provide you with growth opportunities.

How to Use This Book

This book is intended to be a roadmap, and while roadmaps certainly can be read in the moment, if you are at the intersection and do not know which direction to turn, and someone is honking behind you, you may wish you had set your course in advance. So, as you thumb through this book, consider that it contains ample information to be a proactive guide for you, and that it also offers interesting sights to see along the way and hazards to avoid. At the end of each chapter, we suggest points for pondering and provide space for you to make notes. We also encourage you to download the worksheets from Heather's website (www.heatherbrod.com) to help you navigate your journey. You are also welcome to reproduce and share them, but we kindly request proper citation.

We have drawn on our personal experiences, and those of our colleagues and coaching clients, to present a wide range of experiences and multiple perspectives to handle the big questions that arise throughout the course of one's career.

Ultimately, our goal is that you will be imbued with awareness of your environment and armed with self-knowledge to make the best choices for you at any given point in your career. In other words, this is not about determining the shortest route between two points but providing the most unique and beneficial way to get closer to your destination. We strongly believe that the journey is its own reward and that knowledge is power.

This book is not intended to be an epic scholarly tome, addressing how to do research or how to be a better teacher or clinician. There are ample resources that cover these aspects of developing an academic career, such as Roberts' *The Academic Medicine Handbook: A Guide to Achievement and Fulfillment for Academic Faculty* [2]. In Roberts' nearly 500-page book, you'll learn from a wide array of experts about: approaching the profession of academic medicine; getting established; approaching work with colleagues; writing and evaluating manuscripts; conducting empirical research; developing administrative skills; advancing your academic career; and balancing professional and personal life. We highly recommend this valuable resource. However, our vision is that this book will serve as a means to help you define and navigate *your* path in academic medicine.

It is our sincere hope that this book will be a roadmap for your academic success, ensuring that you won't get lost. We want you to have a thriving career in academic medicine. We know how hard it can be and we know how rewarding it can be. We know the success strategies to employ and the landmines to avoid. This book endeavors to address all of the things that a faculty member *really* needs to know to be successful in a concise yet comprehensive guide.

References and Sources

1. The Association of American Medical Colleges (AAMC). https://www.aamc.org/about-us. Accessed 5 Mar 2024.
2. Roberts LW, editor. The academic medicine handbook: a guide to achievement and fulfillment for academic faculty. New York: Springer; 2013.
3. Callanan CJ, Bruder M, Skarupski KA. Faculty factory: snippets for success. June 2021. https://facultyfactory.org/ebook#snippet. Accessed 5 Mar 2024.
4. Callahan CJ, Skarupski KA. Faculty factory: habits and hacks from Hopkins (H^3). June 2022. https://facultyfactory.org/ebook#habits. Accessed 5 Mar 2024.
5. Covey SR. The 7 habits of highly effective people. Simon & Schuster; 2020.
6. Skarupski KA. The FacultyFactory website. Johns Hopkins Medicine. https://facultyfactory.org/. Accessed 5 Mar 2024.
7. Skarupski KA The Faculty Factory podcast. Johns Hopkins Medicine. https://facultyfactory.org/podcast/. Accessed 5 Mar 2024.
8. Skarupski KA. The Faculty Factory podcast Youtube channel. Johns Hopkins Medicine. https://www.youtube.com/channel/UCG6e2L882-m1ARXNK05gKow/playlists?view_as=subscriber. Accessed 5 Mar 2024.
9. Farrell TW, Greer AG, Bennie S, Hageman H, Pfeifle A. Academic health centers and the quintuple aim of health care. Acad Med. 2023;98(5):563–8.
10. Writing Accountability Groups (WAGs) website. https://www.wagyourwork.com/. Accessed 5 Mar 2024.

Acknowledgments

To our faculty affairs and faculty development colleagues:
How many times have you thought, *I wish there was a book that I could give my faculty to help them know what is really important and aid their growth?* We hope that this is it and that it will make your lives just a little bit easier. We envision your ability to annotate this book with the specific resources and key contacts at your institutions to personalize this for your faculty members.

We feel extremely fortunate to be part of a strong collegial group of professionals who dedicate themselves to the growth and development of others. The benefits we have received through your collaboration and partnership are huge and it is a pleasure to give something in return.

Heather's Acknowledgments

My professional journey has been influenced and shaped by many people, though none more so than Robert "Bob" Bornstein, PhD. His guidance and mentorship are evident on every page I have written. In 2009, he hired me as a program manager and encouraged me to make the job my own. He often said that it was his job to open doors, but my job to walk through them. And he opened a lot of doors, providing ample opportunity for continuous growth, learning, and development. The most significant opportunity came in 2010 when he invited me to join a small group of respected colleagues to create a center for faculty development. Despite my lack of experience in talent or organizational development and my limited knowledge of faculty career progression, I embraced the opportunity.

It was through this experience that I discovered talents hidden within myself, grew my confidence, and with Bob's expert guidance, learned how to navigate organizational complexities. He consistently taught me how to think rather than what to think, shaping my ability to generalize learning and apply it across disciplines, which culminated in the creation of the Center for Faculty Advancement, Mentoring and Engagement (FAME) at The Ohio State University's College of Medicine. This experience was singularly transformative, altering my entire trajectory by providing me with skills, knowledge, and expertise that fostered a true career, not just a job. The fulfillment and gratification that Bob helped me find are what I strive to help others discover, as it is incredibly rewarding.

Leading FAME for nearly 10 years, I had the privilege of working with an exceptional team, achieving far more than the sum of our parts. Philip Binkley, MD, and I partnered through it all, with special thanks to the other founders: Kate Dillingham, John Mahan, MD, and Amanda Termuhlen, MD. We were fortunate to collaborate with numerous program directors and contributors, including Anil Agarwal, MD; Amalia Cochran, MD; E. Christopher Ellison, MD; Elizabeth English; Syl Gray; Michael Guertin, MD; Martha Gulati, MD; Larry Hurtubise, PhD; Clara Lee, MD; Mary Mazik; Leon McDougle, MD; Dan McFarlane, MD; Patrick Nana-Sinkam, MD; Tatiana "Tania" Oberyszyn, PhD; Thomas Papadimos, MD; Bhagwan Satiani, MD; Steve Steinberg, MD; Susheela Tridandapani, PhD; Joanne Turner, PhD; David Way; and Karyn Wulf, MD; from whom I learned so much. Thank you.

Special thanks to Aubré Huber, our first hire, for being an insightful thought partner and creating critical infrastructure that effectively supported the ever-expanding mission of faculty development; Debbie Pond for her enthusiastic leadership and can-do attitude, which created a dynamic learning environment; and Emma Tippett for her exceptional data analysis skills, which professionalized our operations and helped us understand our impact on faculty development. Your leadership and contributions were pivotal to shaping the focus, content, and delivery of faculty development, and each of you left an indelible mark on me and FAME.

To all the faculty members I have collaborated with, advised, coached, and mentored—this book would not have been possible without you. From Bob, I learned to ask, "What have you done and why does it matter?" Your struggles to articulate the impact of your work inspired me to write this book. Academic medicine holds immense potential for providing meaningful service *and* deriving personal fulfillment, and my goal is to help everyone who wishes to unlock that potential.

To that end, I am grateful to the Hudson Institute of Coaching for their training, which helped me integrate faculty professional development with principles of adult development. And very special thanks to my small learning groups for supporting and encouraging me during a very difficult period of my life. I wouldn't be on the other side without you.

To my clients who have trusted me with their challenges and dreams, thank you. Your openness and trust have been a privilege. I sometimes think of myself as a pollinator, as I take in insight and wisdom from all of you and spread it around.

To my co-author Kim—thank you! You are truly my sister from another mister. Your energy and collaboration have made this journey wonderful. I am proud of our work and delighted to call you a friend.

To Kevin—I'm incredibly grateful for your love and belief in me. Your support provided the confidence to bet on myself and unlock my golden handcuffs.

Lastly, to our editor and publisher, your guidance and support have been invaluable in bringing this book to fruition. Thank you for believing in our vision.

Kim's Acknowledgments

To all the mentors, colleagues, and professionals from whom I have learned everything I know about faculty affairs and faculty development—Drs.: Denis Evans; Ali Keshavarzian; Susanna Chubinskaya; Janice Clements; Cynthia Rand; Linda Dillon Jones; Barbara Fivush; Jennifer Haythornthwaite; David Yousem; Michael Barone; Rachel Levine; Nauder Faraday; Maria Oliva-Hemker; Jennifer Lee-Summers; and Ms. Laura Robbins; our Association of American Medical Colleges (AAMC) Group on Faculty Affairs (GFA) family; our international Faculty Factory (facultyfactory.org) podcast community; and our WAGs (wagyourwork.com) community—I bow in gratitude—"the divine in me honors the divine in you."

Finally, if you want to write a book, do it with a friend! This book was Heather's idea and we truly had fun volleying it back-and-forth over the interNETs (she doing it tennis-style and I doing it pickleball-style). Heather and I had co-created the Hopkins Career Development Coaching Camp (a weekend retreat for faculty members) and then we needed a new project, hence this book. In addition to Heather being an expert in faculty development and faculty affairs, she's a very deep thinker, a terrific writer, and is simply the best coach I know.

Contents

1	Why Academic Medicine?	1
2	Preparing for an Academic Medicine Career	7
3	Who Am I?	11
4	Getting the Right Position in Academic Medicine	17
5	Your First Year(s) in Academic Medicine—Or in a New Role in Academic Medicine	23
6	Minding the "Academic" in Medicine	31
7	Promotion	37
8	Leadership	43
9	What to Do When (Not if) Things Get Rough	49
10	Infusing Diversity into Your Work and Embracing an Inclusive Mindset	57
11	The Work-Life Integration Paradox	61
12	Transitions	65
Index		71

About the Authors

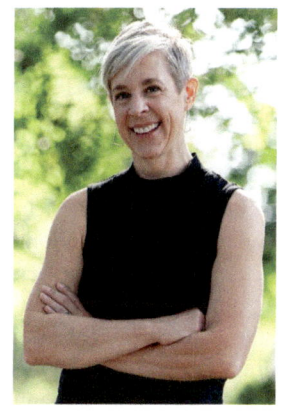

Heather Brod, MA is an executive coach, consultant, speaker, and facilitator primarily to the higher education, healthcare, and professional services industries. As a coach, she helps professionals cultivate mindsets and habits of authentic leadership. As a consultant, she works with companies to create and implement inclusive strategies that develop and leverage the skills of the workforce.

She is a nationally recognized expert in career development and has designed and delivered countless workshops and presentations on topics encompassing diversity, equity, and inclusion, employee retention, culturally responsive mentoring practices, and models for career development.

For over a decade, Heather led an organizational and talent development center for The Ohio State University's College of Medicine. She co-founded the Midwest Collaborative for Faculty Affairs and Development (MCFAD), was a 2019 recipient of Ohio State's Glass Breaker Award, and is Past-President of the Columbus Chapter of the Healthcare Businesswomen's Association.

Heather earned her coaching certification from the Hudson Institute of Coaching and is accredited as a Professional Certified Coach by the International Coaching Federation. She has made Columbus, Ohio, her home for over 20 years (https://www.linkedin.com/in/heather-brod-81b3784/, heather@heatherbrod.com).

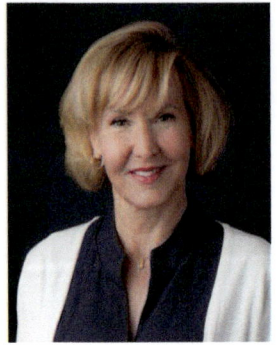

Kimberly Skarupski, PhD, MPH is the Associate Vice Provost for Leadership Development in the Office of Faculty Affairs at the University of Texas Medical Branch at Galveston, Texas. She is also Professor of Internal Medicine - Geriatrics in the John Sealy School of Medicine, and Professor of Epidemiology in the School of Public and Population Health. Formerly, Dr. Skarupski was the Senior Associate Dean for Faculty Development at Johns Hopkins University in Baltimore, MD.

The goal throughout Dr. Skarupski's 17-year faculty development career has been to "build community" (e.g., Writing Accountability Groups [WAGs]; Grant Review Investigator Groups; Specific Aims Speed Sessions; Late-Career and "Next Chapter" Senior Faculty Transitions; group coaching; and building, evaluation, and teaching in various leadership programs). Kim is a certified professional coach through the College of Executive Coaching and has developed group coaching and career development coaching camps for the Hopkins School of Medicine faculty. Kim hosts the Faculty Factory podcast—an international forum for academic affairs and faculty development conversations and a repository of faculty development snippets for academic medical faculty members. As a social gerontologist and program evaluator, the major theme running throughout Kim's 25+ year research career has been the quality of life in older adults, using data from large-scale epidemiologic studies to examine disparities in quality of life, as well as the contribution of various social and psychological determinants of quality of life in older age. Most recently, she has merged her gerontologic and faculty development interests exploring late-career faculty members': career needs; retirement expectations and experiences; and caregiving roles (kskarupski@gmail.com).

Chapter 1
Why Academic Medicine?

It is interesting that you won't find "Academic Medicine" in Wikipedia. You'll get a redirect to "Medicine"—it's branches and history, but the word "Academic" never appears in the entry. Wikipedia will tell you that "Medicine is the science and practice of caring for a patient, managing the diagnosis, prognosis, prevention, treatment, palliation of their injury or disease, and promoting their health." A quick Bing search for "Academic Medicine" points you to the premier journal in the field, called Academic Medicine and you might also run across reference to a *British Medical Journal* article [1] defining academic medicine as a "loosely defined term which describes the branch of medicine pursued by doctors who engage in a variety of scholarly activities."

However, a search of "academic health centers" (AHCs) will get you to the Alliance of Academic Health Centers where you'll read that "an academic health center encompasses all the health-related components of *universities*. It has, or has among its partners, a *school* of medicine, one or more additional health professions *schools*, and/or advanced medical research programs, and a relationship to one or more *teaching* hospitals or health systems." You will notice in this definition that the words: *universities*, *school(s)*, *and teaching* are associated with academic health. Academic health centers are often directly affiliated with schools of medicine and allied health professions.

Academic medicine stands apart from other types of healthcare through its unique integration of medical education, clinical care, research, and community engagement. To understand academic medicine, it is helpful to view it in relation to community healthcare. Academic health centers are positioned at the forefront of medical advancements and innovation, whereas community hospitals play a crucial role in providing essential healthcare services to the local population. Community hospitals focus primarily on delivering primary healthcare services, offering a range

© The Author(s), under exclusive license to Springer Nature
Switzerland AG 2024
H. Brod, K. Skarupski, *The Insider's Pocket Guide to Navigating a Faculty Career in Academic Medicine*, https://doi.org/10.1007/978-3-031-66096-2_1

of medical care that includes general medicine, pediatrics, and obstetrics. The emphasis is on accessible care and ensuring comprehensive healthcare delivery.

Whereas providing clinical care is a shared element across healthcare settings, academic medicine often involves a higher level of specialization and access to the latest treatments. Academic medical centers are at the forefront of adopting new medical technologies and therapies, ensuring that patients receive the most advanced care available. Faculty members in academic medicine are encouraged to stay current with the latest medical advancements, contributing to evidence-based practices and aligning patient care with the latest research findings. As such, continuing professional development is critical.

A primary distinguishing feature of academic medicine is the central role of teaching. Faculty members actively engage in instructing medical students, residents, and fellows, contributing significantly to the training of the next generation of healthcare professionals. In the academic medicine environment, multidisciplinary collaboration thrives. Healthcare professionals, researchers, and educators collaborate closely to address complex medical issues, leading to comprehensive and innovative approaches to patient care and research.

Research and innovation form another unique aspect of academic medicine. Faculty members are deeply involved in a spectrum of research activities, ranging from basic science to clinical trials. This commitment to research helps advance medical knowledge and introduces cutting-edge therapies and technologies, distinguishing academic medical centers as leaders in medical science.

Furthermore, academic medical centers play a role in community engagement. They often participate in community health outreach and education, addressing public health issues, promoting preventive care, and contributing to the overall well-being of the broader community. This multifaceted approach sets academic medicine apart as an environment where healthcare professionals serve not only as practitioners but also as educators and researchers, actively contributing to the advancement of medical knowledge and improved patient outcomes.

Aims. Another way of thinking about academic medicine is its aims. In 2008, the triple aim (*care, health, and cost*) was introduced [2]: to improve the individual experience of care for patients; improve the health of populations; and reduce the per capita cost of care. In 2014, on the heels of burnout in healthcare, a fourth aim was proposed—*care of the health care provider* [3]. Most recently, a fifth aim debuted—*justice* [4]. Hence, a career in academic medicine necessitates a commitment to quintuple aims: patient care; population health; cost of care; provider care; and health equity and justice.

Faculty: The word "faculty" is uniquely associated with academia, implying "a fundamental academic component to one's professional roles and responsibilities;" indeed, "active scholarship is considered essential to the success of all faculty members" [5, 6, p. 280]. Whereas in the past, clinician scientists were known as "triple threats" because they excelled as educators, scholars and clinicians; today, the increase in specialization and change in payment models means that while most individuals engage in all parts of the academic mission, they have a primary focus in one area. Thus, you might see designations like, "clinician investigator," "clinician educator," "educator investigator," etc.

While most physicians are faculty, not all faculty are physicians. There are also scientists, epidemiologists, psychologists, physical therapists, sociologists, bioethicists and many other medical specialists who comprise the faculty of a school of medicine. The critical differentiator of faculty members is their service as educators and scholars. They design and deliver educational content, facilitate clinical experiences, mentor learners in the lab, and otherwise contribute to the developing trainees.

Research is a significant component of the faculty role in academic medicine. Faculty members are actively involved in designing and conducting studies, publishing research findings, and contributing to the advancement of medical knowledge. This commitment to research ensures that academic medicine institutions remain at the forefront of scientific discovery and innovation.

Faculty also serve in leadership roles in academic health centers. They often assume roles such as department chairs, division directors, program directors, or leaders of research programs. In these capacities, they provide strategic direction, oversee academic programs, and contribute to the institution's overall mission. Their leadership extends beyond administrative responsibilities, influencing the culture of collaboration and excellence within the broader academic community.

Faculty roles in academic medicine have changed rather dramatically over the past few decades. As the concept of tenure (*an indefinite academic appointment*) becomes increasingly outdated, physicians within academic medical centers (AMCs) find themselves lacking the job security enjoyed by their predecessors. Many physicians are now employed under contractual agreements with periodic renewals, ranging from annual to every 5 years, among other durations, at the discretion of the AMC. Similarly, termination clauses in contracts allow for employment to be terminated at any time, based on business decisions or at the discretion of the institution. Job security concerns, particularly among early-career physicians, are exacerbated by the lack of a clear academic roadmap for success. Addressing these concerns is crucial not only to mitigate burnout but also to fulfill the fundamental need for job security among physicians.

A career in academic medicine will indeed enrich your intellectual bank account, but not necessarily your financial bank account. You will definitely earn more money if you go into private practice, and you also won't be expected to teach or do research. Thus, as Kingston and Behjati [1] state: "…unless you are willing to commit yourself to your career and to put in those extra hours, academic medicine is not for you." Indeed, as a clinician scientist or basic science researcher, a successful career in academic medicine is built on extraordinarily hard work, dedication, and resilience. Via the Association of American Medical College's (AAMC) annual faculty salary report, you can learn the salary ranges for academic medicine faculty based on region of the country, private or public institution, by degree type (MD or PhD—in clinical or basic sciences), academic rank, department, gender, and race/ethnicity. You can gain access to the report in your school of medicine leadership offices or libraries.

So if the takeaway thus far is that you get to work harder and make less money, you may be asking yourself, why on earth would I want to have a career in academic medicine? Choosing a career in academic medicine is choosing an inspiring journey with a profound sense of purpose and fulfillment. It goes beyond the routine aspects of clinical practice, providing an opportunity to contribute to something bigger than yourself, something that is meaningful and lasting. In academic medicine, you can find joy in shaping the future of healthcare, influencing the trajectory of medical education, and actively participating in groundbreaking research. It's about making a tangible impact on individual patient outcomes and on the broader landscape of medical knowledge and community health. This career path allows you to leave a meaningful legacy and make a lasting difference in the field of healthcare.

Points to Ponder
- What appeals to me about academic medicine? What doesn't appeal to me?
- What kind of contribution to medicine do I want to make?
- What are my thoughts about research and teaching?
- What do I need to learn more about with respect to having a career in academic medicine?

Notes
_____
_____
_____

References

1. Kingston O, Behjati S. Academic medicine. BMJ. 2008;336:s172. https://doi.org/10.1136/bmj.39576.631238.CE.
2. Berwick DM, Nolan TW, Whittington J. The triple aim: care, health, and cost. Health Affairs (Millwood). 2008;27(3):759–69.

3. Bodenheimer T, Sinsky C. From triple to quadruple aim: care of the patient requires care of the provider. Ann Fam Med. 2014;12(6):573–6.
4. Farrell TW, Greer AG, Bennie S, Hageman H, Pfeifle A. Academic health centers and the quintuple aim of health care. Acad Med. 2023;98(5):563–8. https://doi.org/10.1097/ACM.0000000000005031.
5. Bellini LM, Kaplan B, Fischel JE, Meltzer C, Peterson P, Sonnino RE. The definition of faculty must evolve: a call to action. Acad Med. 2020;95(10):1515–20.
6. Block SM, Sonnino RE, Bellini L. Defining "faculty" in academic medicine: responding to the challenges of a changing environment. Acad Med. 2015;90(3):279–82.

Further Readings

AAMC. Group on Faculty Affairs (GFA) Leadership Guide for Faculty Affairs Professionals. https://www.aamc.org/career-development/affinity-groups/gfa/leadership-guide-faculty-affairs-professionals. Accessed 27 Feb 2024.
AAMC. https://www.aamc.org/data-reports/workforce/report/aamc-faculty-salary-report. Accessed 27 Feb 2024.
Alliance of Academic Health Centers. Member Benefits. "What is an academic health center?" https://www.aamc.org/media/66306/download?attachment. Accessed 27 Feb 2004.
Association of American Medical Colleges (AAMC). Faculty Roster: U.S. Medical School Faculty. Trends. https://www.aamc.org/data-reports/faculty-institutions/report/faculty-roster-us-medical-school-faculty. Accessed 27 Feb 2024.
Collins RT 2nd, Sanford R. The importance of formalized, lifelong physician career development: making the case for a paradigm shift. Acad Med. 2021;96(10):1383–8. https://doi.org/10.1097/ACM.0000000000004191.
Medscape Physician Compensation Report, 2022. https://www.medscape.com/slideshow/2022-compensation-overview-6015043?reg=1#2. Accessed 27 Feb 2024.
Shanafelt TD, Hasan O, Dyrbye LN, Sinsky C, Satele D, Sloan J, West CP. Changes in burnout and satisfaction with work-life balance in physicians and the general US working population between 2011 and 2014. Mayo Clin Proc. 2015;90(12):1600–13.
West CP, Dyrbye LN, Shanafelt TD. Physician burnout: contributors, consequences, and solutions. J Intern Med. 2018;283(6):516–29.
Wikipedia. https://en.wikipedia.org/wiki/Medicine#Institutions. Accessed 27 Feb 2024.

Chapter 2
Preparing for an Academic Medicine Career

If you are still in the phase of your training where you are considering whether you want an academic career, you'll want to get serious about the "academic" part. What does that mean exactly? It means that as an academic, you are expected to excel at teaching and scholarship, in addition to your clinical and research work, so it is important to set your course so that you can gain experience doing academic work throughout your training.

A useful framework is Boyer's classification of scholarship [1], introduced by Ernest Boyer in 1990, which delineates four dimensions of scholarship: discovery, integration, application, and teaching. In the context of academic medicine, this framework demonstrates that the nature of scholarly activity extends beyond what we would consider "traditional" research. It recognizes the value of generating new knowledge (discovery), integrating diverse sources of information, applying knowledge to solve real-world problems, and effectively communicating insights through teaching and mentorship. For medical professionals, this model encourages engagement in a broader spectrum of scholarly endeavors, including clinical innovation, curriculum development, and community outreach, fostering a culture of continuous learning and improvement within the field.

Faculty in academia enjoy the "*academic freedom*" to pursue their own interests; however, academic freedom comes with academic responsibility. Responsibilities as an academic faculty member include the faithful execution of professional duties and obligations in adherence to your institution's academic policies and procedures. Expect that professional duties will include practicing your trade (as an MD, PhD, ScD, other professional degree) *and* being an 'academic'—meaning an educator and a scholar. That is, in academic medicine, faculty members very rarely spend 100% of their effort seeing patients or doing research. If you're an MD, you will split your time between: clinical practice; research; teaching, program building; and service to your division or department, school, institution, and community on various committees, task forces, working groups, boards, etc. If you're a PhD, you will similarly split your time between: research; teaching; program building; and the same service roles as above. Whatever you're doing, you will be held accountable to having local, regional, national, and, at the professorial level, international impact in your field(s).

Faculty in academic medicine are scholars who engage in rigorous research endeavors aimed at addressing critical questions within the medical field. This involves conducting clinical trials, observational studies, or basic science research to expand our understanding of diseases, treatment modalities, and healthcare systems. Scholars publish their findings, thereby contributing to the broader scientific community and influencing medical practices. Various types of scholars contribute to the diverse landscape of research, education, and clinical practice. These scholars often specialize in specific roles that align with their interests, expertise, and career goals. Some prominent types of scholars in academic medicine include clinician-scientists, basic scientists, medical educators, and healthcare policy researchers.

Clinician-scientists form a vital category of scholars in academic medicine. These individuals actively engage in both clinical practice and scientific research, combining their expertise to bridge the gap between laboratory discoveries and patient care. Clinician-scientists often conduct translational research, seeking to apply scientific insights to the development of innovative medical treatments and interventions. Their dual roles as practitioners and researchers allow them to bring a unique perspective to both the laboratory and the clinic.

Basic scientists are the foundation of biomedical research; they study the fundamental biological processes and causal mechanisms of health and illness and conduct 'bench science' to test their hypotheses. Basic scientists work in biological chemistry, biomedical engineering, biophysics and biophysical chemistry, molecular and comparative pathobiology, cell biology, molecular biology and genetics, neuroscience, pharmacology and molecular sciences, physiology, and the like. Their discoveries inform diagnoses, treatments, cures, and prevention of diseases and solutions to maximize health.

Medical educators are another essential group of scholars who focus on shaping the next generation of healthcare professionals. These scholars are dedicated to teaching medical students, residents, and fellows, imparting not only clinical knowledge but also instilling critical thinking skills and a commitment to evidence-based practice. They may develop innovative educational approaches, contribute to curriculum design, and engage in scholarly activities related to medical education, ensuring a continuous cycle of learning and improvement.

Healthcare policy researchers in academic medicine focus on understanding and influencing the broader systems and policies that impact healthcare delivery. These scholars may conduct research on healthcare disparities, health economics, and policy interventions aimed at improving population health. By examining the social determinants of health and advocating for policy changes, healthcare policy researchers contribute to shaping the landscape of healthcare delivery and promoting equitable access to medical services.

Each type of scholar in academic medicine brings a unique perspective and skill set, collectively contributing to the advancement of medical knowledge and the improvement of patient outcomes. Additionally, scholars in academic medicine are also deeply involved in teaching and mentoring. They play a pivotal role in educating medical students, residents, and fellows, sharing not only their clinical expertise but also instilling the importance of evidence-based practice and critical thinking. Through mentorship, they guide aspiring healthcare professionals in navigating the complexities of both clinical and research aspects of medicine.

Very few faculty members in academic medicine are specifically taught how to teach or mentor. It is something that most people learn by observing, seeking specific mentorship or guidance, and then self-studying. Therefore, if you are a medical student, resident, fellow, doctoral student or post-doctoral fellow with a passion for teaching, it is wise to invest time in understanding the foundational principles for teaching and education. For example, in the Johns Hopkins University School of Medicine, the Domains of Educators' Work are: teaching and facilitating learning; program and curriculum development; assessment and evaluation; educational leadership; educational scholarship; and educational mentoring, coaching, and advising [2]. Your professors can mentor you about teaching, and reading articles in scholarly education journals in your field helps you to learn the vocabulary and methods of teaching.

In academia, faculty members are promoted through various ranks. Academic ranks vary by institution; but generally, from lowest to highest, faculty ranks are: research associate; instructor, assistant professor, associate professor, and (full) professor. Criteria for promotion always include some indicators of local, national or international impact in the field of practice (e.g., via research funding and peer-reviewed publications or via clinical or educational excellence practice indicators such as patient referrals and testimonials, caseloads, techniques and methods, teaching awards, educational scholarship, visiting lectures, invited presentations, patents, projects and programs, etc.). Tenure, an appointment category that promises 'indefinite employment' (barring extraordinary circumstances), may exist in some academic institutions. That is, in some institutions, if you are "on the tenure track," there are expectations for your performance and scholarly impact. Once you've met those expectations, you may earn promotion to a "tenured appointment"—usually at the associate professor or professor rank. Other institutions may not have tenure per se, but may instead have a "contract to retirement" clause.

In your early years (typically up to 7 years), a team of mentors and sponsors can help support your professional and career development (read more about mentorship in Chap. 5). You will be establishing the networks to build your: research agenda; clinical practice; educational portfolio; program development; and institutional, professional society(ies), and community service roles. You will engage with your office of faculty development to shore-up your knowledge and skills in areas like: how to get promoted; leadership; communication; building relationships; infusing diversity, equity, and inclusion in your work; scholarly- and grant-writing; teaching skills; etc.

By mid-career, you've established a national reputation via your clinical, educational, or research expertise and are likely serving as a mentor to many trainees and early-career faculty members. You will likely be leading division or departmental committees or initiatives and serving on your professional societies' various leadership committees. By mid-career, you may have been given various leadership opportunities and titles (e.g., program director, division director). Later-career, you've established an international reputation, have built a strong: research lab and funding career; a thriving clinical practice or a robust educational reputation; and have trained and mentored numerous early-career faculty members and learners. Later-career faculty members are more likely to hold institutional leadership roles such as division directors or department chairperson or associate deans.

If you are committed to a career in academic medicine, preparation might begin as early as high school, spending summers in a research lab learning and practicing science and writing. I (Kim) hired an administrative coordinator who had graduated college with honors and had three peer-reviewed publications. It turned-out that her college dormitory roommate's father was a neuroradiologist at Hopkins. After she suffered a head injury playing soccer, she became interested in medicine and spent her summer breaks working in his research lab. She knew during that experience that she wanted to be a physician scientist. She told me this during her interview and had her whole life planned. She wanted to work with us to learn more about faculty life, study for her MCATs, get married, have two children, go to medical school, and spend her career in academic medicine. She has done exactly that—in that order. Your path may not be that ordered and linear, but you can appreciate that one must have both a passion for and commitment to medicine and/or science and scholarship.

Points to Ponder
- What kind of scholar do I want to be? What type of knowledge contribution do I want to make?
- What is my interest in teaching?
- What can I do to improve my skills?
- How is my writing habit? What can I do to master my writing skills and routine?

Notes
_____
_____
_____

References

1. Boyer EL, et al. Scholarship reconsidered: priorities of the professoriate. Hoboken: Wiley; 2015.
2. Cofrancesco J, Levine L. Report of the Educator Competencies and Metrics Committee. Baltimore: Johns Hopkins University School of Medicine; 2021.

Further Readings

Skarupski KA. WAG your work: writing accountability groups: bootcamp for increasing scholarly productivity. New York: Amazon Press; 2018.

Skarupski KA, Foucher K. Writing Accountability Groups (WAGs): a tool to help junior faculty members build sustainable writing habits. J Fac Dev. 2018;32(3):47–54.

Chapter 3
Who Am I?

The first chapters may have you feeling a bit overwhelmed. You may be thinking that academic medicine is complex and hard, and that getting to that sweet spot of fulfillment is a pipe dream. The complexity is accurate; however, fulfillment is not a pipe dream. It is entirely possible if you know and trust yourself.

If asked the question, "who are you?" How will you answer? Chances are, you will say something like, "I'm Kim. I am the associate vice provost for leadership development, a researcher, a pickleball player, a dog mom." And yes, that is true; however, those are your roles, the way you present yourself to the outside world, they do not really capture the essence of you—they are merely *what you do, not who you are!* In total, you are more like what Walt Whitman wrote—"you contain multitudes" [1].

You may not realize it, but you have been going through a process of professional identity formation since college, and it was greatly shaped during postgraduate education as you began the specific training for your future career [2]. Couple this with your growth and development as a person, and the result is who you are right now. But don't be fooled into thinking that who you are right now is who you'll be in the future. The "right now" piece is key because you can and will change as you continue to accrue experiences and interact within your profession and the world at large. Interestingly, Quoidbach et al. [3] shed light on the "end of history illusion" through their interviews with 19,000 individuals spanning ages 18–68. Despite respondents acknowledging substantial changes in their past, they collectively believed that their future selves would change relatively little. This phenomenon highlights that we often underestimate the magnitude of future change. Your career may take many interesting turns; your values may shift.

In essence, who you are is a combination of what you do and what you hold to be personally significant, reflecting various qualities, conditions, beliefs, values and ideals. Professional identity is formed by integrating one's professional and personal self, mixing norms and conditions of the profession with a person's own understanding of self [4]. It is easy to think of identity as something that is stable, and for those of us who spend a very long time learning our professions, the profession can take on outsized importance or cause us to shape ourselves around it, instead of being malleable. This is what makes self-awareness and self-knowing so important. They are integrity anchors for decision-making.

Making choices in alignment with who you are creates a greater sense of fulfillment and satisfaction in life. The suggestions we provide in this chapter can be revisited at any time in a career and especially should be considered when major opportunities arise, at significant life events (e.g., marriage, childbirth, promotion, health issues, divorce, death/loss, etc.), and when feelings of dissatisfaction occur. (Refer back here when you read about "What to do when things get rough" in Chap. 9 and "Transitions" in Chap. 11). You will find worksheets and tools that supplement this chapter at Heather's website: www.heatherbrod.com.

There are many ways to deepen self-knowing, and a good starting point is values. Values are at the core of our beliefs and decision-making. Values are comprised of concepts that we hold to be true. They are intimately tied to our aspirations and goals and relate to behaviors that we find desirable. Unlike externally imposed norms or rules, our values transcend particular situations and are instead overarching guiding principles that help us navigate our lives. They shape our actions and reactions, helping us to select and evaluate our behavior and the events around us. We prioritize our values according to their significance in our lives at a particular time.

Consequently, misaligned values are a source of tremendous dissatisfaction. If you find yourself feeling dissatisfied at work, consider that your values may not be aligned with your working culture's values. And note that when we refer to the working culture's values, we refer to the behaviors that the culture rewards, not the organizational values that are stated in the institution's brand. These often differ. Experiencing values misalignment is a path to burnout [5, 6].

It is helpful to identify 5–10 values that reflect who you are in your best incarnation. There are several methods to do this, and in our coaching practices, we find that the process outlined by Mindtools [7] works particularly well. It asks you to reflect on key life moments and then to select values words that most resonate with you from a list, and then to winnow them down through reflection or forced-ranking. In addition, you can find numerous lists of values online, as well as on www.heatherbrod.com (see references).

Assessments are another tool for raising self-awareness. There are thousands of assessments on the market. In our experience, academics have a tendency to over-analyze the validity of the assessment tool, thereby missing the opportunity to gain insight. Our guidance is to view these tools as just that—*tools* to help your brain get curious. Here are some of our preferred tools:

- Gallup, CliftonStrengths [8]: This tool comprises 177 paired statements, allowing you to select the one that best describes you. The result is a ranking of 34 themes that highlights your top talents. This assessment advocates for emphasiz-

ing and leveraging strengths rather than attempting to address weaknesses as the primary path to personal and professional growth.
- Myers-Briggs Type Indicator (MBTI): This personality assessment classifies individuals into one of 16 personality types based on preferences in four dichotomies: extraversion/introversion, sensing/intuition, thinking/feeling, and judging/perceiving. It offers valuable insights into personality traits, communication styles, and decision-making preferences.
- The Enneagram [9]: Categorizing individuals into one of nine personality types based on core motivations, fears, and desires, this assessment provides deep insights for personal growth, self-awareness, and understanding of relationships. It goes beyond the MBTI by delving into the motivations and fears that underlie behavior.
- VIA Character Assessment [10]: Prioritizing an individual's top character strengths from a list of 24, this tool is designed to foster well-being, resilience, and personal growth.
- 360 Assessment: Various tools in the market offer this type of assessment, involving a self-rating compared to feedback from peers, direct reports, and supervisors. This comprehensive approach provides a 360-degree view of how you are perceived as a leader.

Most of these assessments can be found online and sometimes there are free versions (see references). The best results will come from working with a certified professional who can both administer and debrief the assessment with you.

Enhancing self-awareness promotes personal growth while extending to the needs of others as well, with Emotional Intelligence (EI) serving as a particularly valuable framework for this purpose. This refers to the ability to recognize and manage one's own emotions, as well as the emotions of others. It includes the ability to empathize with others, read social cues and build positive relationships. EI theory originates from the science of emotions, whereby emotions are recognized as valuable sources of information that aid us in understanding and navigating our internal and social worlds [11].

Being able to demonstrate EI is becoming increasingly important in professional settings. Research has shown that individuals with high emotional intelligence are more successful in their careers, have better mental and physical health, and enjoy more fulfilling personal relationships. They are better equipped to handle stress, communicate effectively, and solve problems, and are generally more resilient in the face of adversity [12].

There are numerous assessments that can help you identify how emotionally intelligent you are and provide guidance to help you continue to grow. A couple that we like are Psychology Today's online EI assessment [13] and Emotional Intelligence 2.0, an assessment contained within a short book by Travis Bradberry [14].

You might be wondering; what do I do with all this insight I am gaining? Great question! The intent of all of this is that personal and professional development is to expand opportunity, thereby creating a richer life. After all, *"knowing yourself is the beginning of all wisdom" (Aristotle) and Socrates also advised us: "Know Thyself"*

However, as you learn and grow, you may find yourself with an abundance of interesting opportunities. The challenge here is not to overcommit and to choose those that are best aligned with your purpose, which raises the question—how do I know my purpose?

Purpose refers to a sense of direction and meaning in life. It is a deep and underlying motivation that drives an individual towards certain goals and aspirations. Your purpose can be defined as your reason for being, or the unique contribution you want to make in the world. It stems from your interests, passions, values, and beliefs and provides a sense of fulfillment and satisfaction. As you seek to understand your purpose, it is helpful to define your personal vision and mission to guide you [15].

A vision statement defines your desired future state. It represents your aspirations and hopes for the future and provides a clear and inspiring image of what you want to achieve. It is broad in scope and longer-term than a mission statement. A mission statement, then, defines the actions you will take to achieve your vision. It is more specific and shorter-term than a vision statement as it provides a framework for how to achieve the desired future that your vision statement describes.

Some examples of vision statements are:

- To create a world where everyone has access to affordable and high-quality healthcare.
- To conduct research that leads to groundbreaking discoveries in cancer prevention and improves quality of life.
- To be a healthcare leader who advocates for policies that promote health equity and social justice.
- To develop innovative technologies that improve the diagnosis, treatment, and prevention of diabetes.
- To be a leader in my field, driving the development of new knowledge about autoimmune disorders and empowering others to contribute to the advancement of medicine.
- To create a supportive and inclusive learning environment that fosters the intellectual and personal growth of students.
- To build a culture of lifelong learning in medicine, where healthcare professionals are continuously improving their knowledge and skills to better serve the community.

Some examples of mission statements are:

- To foster a culture of respect, compassion, and empathy in the healthcare community by treating my patients with dignity and empathy, advocating for the needs of underrepresented patient populations, and promoting a culture of diversity, equity, and inclusion.
- To collaborate widely with other scientists and healthcare professionals to develop new treatments for cancer that improves the quality of life for patients with cancer and promotes cancer prevention in the broader population.

- To advocate for the health and well-being of my patients and the broader community by staying informed about public health policies and initiatives, and using my voice and expertise to advocate for policies that promote equitable access to healthcare for under-served populations in the US.
- To support and empower my patients by educating them about their health conditions and treatment options, listening to their concerns and needs, and collaborating with them to develop effective treatment plans that align with their goals and values.
- To conduct research with integrity and rigor, always striving for scientific excellence by pursuing novel research questions, developing innovative methodologies, and engaging in rigorous peer-review processes.
- To provide exceptional teaching that challenges and inspires my students by incorporating innovative teaching strategies and leveraging technology to create engaging and interactive learning experiences.

We recommend consulting your vision and mission statements when setting goals and when presented with new opportunities and asking yourself, *"is this aligned with my mission? How does this bring my vision to life?"* If an opportunity does not align, and yet you find yourself excited by it, then it is wise to ask yourself, *"is this still the right vision and mission for me or has something shifted?"* If the answer is that something has shifted, consider rewriting your vision and mission statement.

As professional coaches, we would be remiss if we didn't recommend coaching to guide you on your journey of self-awareness. Unfortunately, in some domains, coaching is viewed as a last resort for "problem" employees and is viewed as remediation, undermining its developmental intent to support clients in maximizing their potential. When implemented as intended, coaching provides personalized attention tailored to your specific needs and goals, along with an objective perspective that helps you overcome obstacles and identify blind spots. Coaching fosters accountability and creates clarity around your goals and desired outcomes.

Through continuous learning and intentional career development, you will gain a deeper understanding of who you are and what truly matters to you, ultimately contributing to the unfolding narrative of your purpose in both personal and professional domains. As you acquire new skills and expertise, you will find new avenues to contribute meaningfully to your profession and community. The sense of purpose deepens as you realize the impact of your work on others and society at large. Self-awareness thus is not only about personal growth but also a means to contribute positively to the world, aligning your identity with a broader sense of purpose.

Points to Ponder
- What are my values and how are my actions aligned to my values?
- How do I exhibit emotional intelligence?
- What is my vision, mission and purpose?
- Are my choices and decisions aligned with my purpose, vision and mission?
- How can I deepen my understanding of self?

Notes

_____
_____
_____

References

1. Whitman W. Song of myself. East Aurora: Roycrofters; 1894.
2. Sarraf-Yazdi S, et al. A scoping review of professional identity formation in undergraduate medical education. J Gen Intern Med. 2021;36:3511–21.
3. Quoidbach J, Gilbert DT, Wilson TD. The end of history illusion. Science. 2013;339:96–8. www.sciencemag.org
4. Hitlin S. Values as the core of personal identity: drawing links between two theories of self. Soc Psychol Quart. 2003;66(2):118–37. https://doi.org/10.2307/1519843. Accessed 23 Apr 2023.
5. Begun R. The connection between values and burnout. https://rachelbegun.com/blogposts/the-connection-between-values-and-burnout. Accessed 27 Nov 2023.
6. Shanafelt T. Physician burnout: stop blaming the individual. https://www.youtube.com/watch?v=z9BEfsJOhUY. Accessed 5 Mar 2024.
7. Mindtools. What are your values?: deciding what's important in life, https://www.mindtools.com/a5eygum/what-are-your-values. Accessed 15 Jan 2024.
8. Buckingham M, Clifton DO. Now, discover your strengths. New York: Simon and Schuster; 2001.
9. Riso DR, Hudson R. Understanding the enneagram: the practical guide to personality types. Boston: Houghton Mifflin Harcourt; 2000.
10. Via Institute on Character. https://www.viacharacter.org/. Accessed 5 Mar 2024.
11. Goleman D, Boyatzis RE. https://hbr.org/2017/02/emotional-intelligence-has-12-elements-which-do-you-need-to-work-on.
12. Salovey P, Grewal D. The science of emotional intelligence. Curr Dir Psychol Sci. 2005;14:281–5.
13. Psychology Today, Emotional Intelligence Test. https://www.psychologytoday.com/ca/tests/personality/emotional-intelligence-test. Accessed 15 Jan 2024.
14. Bradberry T, Greaves J. Emotional intelligence 2.0. San Diego: TalentSmart; 2009.
15. Kroth M, Boverie P. Life mission and adult learning. Adult Educ Q. 2000;50(2):134–49.

Further Readings

16 Personalities. https://www.16personalities.com/. Accessed 17 Jan 2024.
Brown B. Dare to lead list of values. https://brenebrown.com/resources/dare-to-lead-list-of-values/.
Center for Creative Leadership. Values explorer card deck. https://shop.ccl.org/usa/values-explorer-card-deck.html.
Dweck C. Growth mindset: the new psychology of success. New York: Ballantine Books; 2007.
Kaufman SB. Transcend: the new science of self-actualization. New York: TarcherPerigee; 2020.
Leider R. The power of purpose: find meaning, live longer, better. San Francisco: Berrett-Koehler Publishers; 2015.
Palmer P. Let your life speak: listening for the voice of vocation. San Francisco: Jossey-Bass; 1999.

Chapter 4
Getting the Right Position in Academic Medicine

The right position for you is subjective. The right job for you will not only feel like "a good fit" but will feel like you *belong* because your values are aligned with the institution's values. Your right position may be in a rural teaching hospital serving people who don't have easy access to or availability of care. Or your right position may be in an academic medical center in a major metropolitan area. Or maybe you want to choose a geographic area because you like the climate, the cost of living, the food or sports culture, or because you want to be closer to family. How will you know where to go?

You need to figure out *what* you should do and *where* you should do it. Of the two questions—what and where—*what* is probably easier. You likely have a pretty good idea of *what* you want to do, based on your specialty or practice area. However, there are many "hidden" considerations within even that. For instance, how much time do you prefer to spend in clinical practice or teaching? If you are a clinician, do you want to practice in an environment that offers a lot of autonomy, or do you want to have a lot of practice partners to share the load? What is the call schedule like? If you are early in your career, what kind of mentorship is important to you? I (Kim) focused my sociology doctoral studies on gerontology and epidemiology because I envisioned myself teaching gerontology at a university *somewhere* and conducting research. The *somewhere* was the primary consideration. Fortunately for me, shortly after I was finishing the first year of my post-doctoral fellowship, a faculty position in a gerontology program nearby became available. Everything aligned; the university was great, the gerontology program was well-respected with renowned faculty members, there was opportunity to grow and build, and it was nearby.

It was fortunate that this position fit into the overall type of life I wanted to have. Your next position doesn't have to be your last position, but you should consider how you want your life to look and feel at least for the next few years. Are you ready to settle-down in the suburbs and be soccer parents? If so, what type of position will support that? And what else will you need to bring this vision to fruition? Proximity to family? On-site daycare? Or maybe you want to pay-down your student loans as fast as possible, so you want maximum volume and low cost-of-living. What type of locale and environment best supports that? Also beware the path of least resistance; that is, accepting a position at your current institution without exploring what other options are available to you or considering the life you want to have now.

Once you're pretty clear on the types of qualities that you would like in an academic medical position, you can begin to assemble a short-list of academic medical centers. You'll find that the number of opportunities you discover will be directly proportional to the size of your network. Your professors, mentors, preceptors, fellow society members, and friends will tell you about great schools, programs, and job openings; return the favor! Social media (LinkedIn, Instagram, Facebook) is increasingly used to job hunt and popular search engines for higher education include the AAMC CareerConnect [1], The Chronicle of Higher Education jobs site [2], and HigherEdJobs [3].

Then, do a lot of research on the institution, the department, and the faculty. All academic medical centers (AMCs)/academic health centers (AHCs) have lovely mission, vision, and values statements; your investigative lens should get you curious about how they actually live their stated values. Try to find the evidence for *how* they live those values. For example, if they value diversity, what proportion of their students, faculty, and leaders are 'diverse'? If they value community, how do they value their faculty and staff members' time actually serving in the community? If they value people, how do they compensate and recognize the extra efforts of their faculty and staff?

Ask your mentors and colleagues what they know about the institution and the faculty members there. Ask your mentors and colleagues to e-introduce you to faculty members and/or trainees there. Ask curious questions of the people who work in the institution you're considering. For example, how many faculty members join the department each year? How many depart? How long do the staff stay? How many staff vacancies are there? Where are the opportunities for improvement? How does the institution demonstrate its commitment to X, Y, or Z?

Prior to applying for a job, Assemble your curriculum vitae in a logical order (get a template from your current institution, use the AAMC's terrific template [4], or simply copy the formatting of a trusted faculty member) and write a compelling introductory letter. Get your list of references prepared; ask mentors for their permission before you list them. Prepare samples of your writing (e.g., the PDFs or links to select manuscripts). Consider hiring a coach who will help you prepare for your initial interview, and then your subsequent on-campus interview. A coach will also help you negotiate for the position and be invaluable in helping you to think about all the resources and items you will need in your start-up package.

Make sure you've done your homework well in advance of your visit. In addition to assessing for values alignment, some things you might want to learn about are: the institution's strategic plan; who the leaders are and how long they have been there; basic information about the department and its national reputation; faculty members' reputations; turnover; students; endowments and other private and philanthropic support; public support at the state (if applicable); research facilities and grants management infrastructure; professional development offerings; the school of medicine's relationship with the hospital and university; governance; funds flow; and their engagement with and reputation in the community. This tells you about the stability of the institution and the types of resources that will be available to you to do what you are hired to do.

Ask the *newest* faculty members at the institution to describe their average work week. Ask them how their research and scholarship is progressing. What support and resources do they have to do their jobs and achieve their goals? What are their major hurdles and hassles? Who is the most successful there and how are they doing it? Are these the kind of people you want to be at your side for the next several years? Assess—do your values align? Do the faculty even know each other, and anything about each other's lives?

Learn about the faculty tracks and what this specific role entails. These determine the basic expectations of your job, such as the allocation of time in teaching, research and service. For instance, if one of your primary responsibilities will be conducting research but the faculty track you're on comes with 80% clinical time, does that allow sufficient time to write grants and meet the expectations for scholarship on which you will eventually be evaluated at promotion time? If you are being asked to start a new clinic or develop a new program, what is needed to launch that? How will your success be measured?

There are different uses of nomenclature for faculty tracks, but some basics are:

- Tenure Track: this is the original academic track, most often granted to "traditional" scholars such as basic science researchers and sometimes clinician-scientists. Some institutions have done away with tenure, others have time-limited tenure appointments. Faculty on the tenure track are expected to engage in all mission areas, though teaching in colleges of medicine is often significantly less than in colleges of arts & sciences, for instance. Conducting NIH-funded research and publishing are the primary expectations of this track.
- Clinical Track: these are typically contract based appointments and may also be described in sub-types, such as clinician-educator or clinician-scholar, denoting the primary emphasis of the appointment. Faculty on this track are expected to engage in all missions to varying degrees. Most physician faculty are hired on a clinical track and clinical service expectations typically will be in excess of 60% of the appointment.
- Research Track (or non-tenure science track): these are usually contract appointments granted to basic scientists with little expectation to produce work beyond conducting research, obtaining grants and publishing manuscripts.
- Adjunct, Auxiliary or Practice Track: these are usually short-term contract appointments, and often not considered part of the "regular" faculty. That is, these appointments are secondary and granted for a specific purpose, such as to teach one course, or to be 100% clinical without expectation of scholarship or teaching. They offer the least protection and fewest faculty rights.

Once you're there, notice the culture. Culture is 'how we do things around here.' What is the tone or vibe? Is it tense or relaxed, noisy or quiet, gloomy or inspiring? Notice not only what people say but what they don't say (i.e., one of our colleagues advises to *be wary of the vagueness of denial*, in other words, learn to listen between the lines). For example, try to gauge how long have people been there. What is the faculty exit rate and why did the most recent people leave? What is the promotion rate, promotion pathways, and promotion criteria? Who in the department was promoted most recently? Can you meet with them and inquire about the process? What resources are there to do your job (e.g., administrative support, pre- and post-awards staff, clinic staff)? What are the expectations of you? Who will mentor you and what does "mentorship" look like for them? How will your work be evaluated?

Importantly, remember that an interview is a two-way street. It is not a process done to you, you are as much assessing and evaluating your desire to be there as they are assessing whether they want you there. Do not be afraid to ask questions. In addition to the practical suggestions above, a good question to ask is, *"can you tell me about how we would work together?"* Finally, trust your gut. If it doesn't feel right, check-in with yourself to attempt to understand why. And even if you can't pinpoint it, if you have a sense of discomfort or unease, it is not the right place for you, no matter its reputation or what is being offered.

You Got an Offer! Congratulations! Now Negotiate!

Regardless of your gender, there is a good book to read before you accept a job: Ask for it [5]. It was written for women, but the tenets are applicable across the board. Almost all employers expect you to negotiate your job offer—almost all! Naturally, most people focus on the salary. Of course, you did your research about salary when you began exploring job opportunities, using Glassdoor, the AAMC's faculty salary data, or by searching public institutions' salary data. Salary is the most obvious negotiating lever because it determines your future earnings (the law of compound interest). Additionally, your pension is based on your annual salary, as is annual cost-of-living adjustments and any future raises that are associated with promotion and leadership opportunities. For physicians, there may be three parts of your salary—Part A may be your baseline salary, Part B is your supplemental salary associated with your clinical practice, and Part C may be a portion of your salary associated with leadership roles in the department or school. Be sure you understand all aspects of your salary, and bonus and raise potential. If you are required to bring in extramural grant funding, understand what percentage of your salary is required to be covered by funding, what type of funding "counts" and by when.

In addition to salary, understand the amount of "protected" time you are being given for research, teaching or administrative work. You also need to understand your faculty rank at hire and the promotion criteria for your desired pathway to ensure that the time and resources you are being given align to those expectations. Then, there are many other negotiable aspects of a position, including: administrative support; office space; research lab space; clinic days; block time; types of programs to be developed; on-call requirements; specific teaching assignments; relocation expenses; equipment; supplies; start-up funds; technology and computers; discounted cell phone service; parking; meals; paid time off (PTO); or gym membership. Don't make any assumptions. For example, you might think that as a faculty member, you'll obviously get an office. But we know faculty members who found themselves sharing a cubicle with three other faculty members. Also, do you have a partner or spouse who would need a job if you relocate? Some institutions have dual-hire processes or will help your partner find a job in the area.

What are your non-negotiables? Have a list and know them. How do you know what those are? Go back to your core values. These represent what is most important to you and if sacrificed will likely result in disappointment. It can be really hard to trust your self-knowing, especially when you are negotiating your first job. However, only you can know what you need and want, and what you need and want may be different from classmates and other colleagues. This is OK! And you can also assess by talking to your friends and colleagues who may be one rung above you on the career ladder and asking them what *they* wish they had known before they signed on the dotted line. Are they doing the things they love?

Whatever you negotiate, make sure it is in writing. Conversations, text messages, even emails won't hold water compared to explicit language in your offer letter. For all practical purposes, if it isn't in your offer letter (or is a written policy of the institution), it doesn't exist. The offer letter will likely undergo at least a couple modifications; make sure you triple-check each version to verify that everything you already agreed to stays in the revisions and nothing else was added without your knowledge. We know of colleagues who signed renegotiated offer letters that they hadn't scrutinized after multiple revisions and discovered changes after the fact. Also know that institutions are concerned with protecting their interests. It's not personal, it's business. Therefore, if you find yourself with a densely legal document that you're being asked to sign, you may consider hiring an attorney to review and explain the consequences of any clauses or provisions, so you know exactly what you are signing.

Points to Ponder
- What qualities are important to me when considering integrating a job and my life?
- Where would I like to live? Or where do I not want to live?
- Who do I know who works at the institution that I'm applying to, or used to work there?
- What are my non-negotiables? What will I negotiate for?
- Where can I find a job coach?
- When considering an offer, do the expectations and offered resources match? What does my gut say?

Notes

References

1. AAMC CareerConnect: connecting talent with opportunities in academic medicine. https://careerconnect.aamc.org/. Accessed 27 Feb 2024.
2. The Chronicle of Higher Education. Jobs. https://jobs.chronicle.com/jobs/. Accessed 27 Feb 2024.
3. HigherEdJobs. https://www.higheredjobs.com/ Accessed 27 Feb 2024.
4. AAMC Preparing your Curriculum Vitae. https://www.aamc.org/professional-development/affinity-groups/gfa/faculty-vitae/preparing-your-curriculum-vitae/. Accessed 27 Feb 2024.
5. Babcock L, Laschever S. Ask for it: how women can use the power of negotiation to get what they really want. New York: Bantam Dell; 2009.

Further Reading

American Association of University Professors (AAUP). Tenure. https://www.aaup.org/issues/tenure#:~:text=What%20is%20academic%20tenure%3F,financial%20exigency%20and%20program%20discontinuation. Accessed 27 Feb 2024.

Chapter 5
Your First Year(s) in Academic Medicine— Or in a New Role in Academic Medicine

Whew! You negotiated a great offer for this stage in your life, and now you are ready to hit the ground running! The question is, which direction? This chapter is intended to help you avoid running in circles by getting to know your environment, the people, how you fit into the picture, and how to establish yourself. This chapter is all about developing your presence at your home institution. No matter where you are in your career, if you have changed institutions, or even taken on a new role in your current institution, these tactics will help you grow and thrive.

When you are brand new to a career in academic medicine, you are likely to feel overwhelmed and even lost. You have spent years training and being told what to do and now suddenly you are on your own. That is why our goal for this book is to demonstrate mindsets so that you can make the best decisions for *you and you alone*. In Chap. 3 (Who am I?), we suggested you spend some deep-thinking time getting to the heart of your values, strengths, purpose, vision, and mission. When you are truly grounded in who you are, it's easier to trust yourself and articulate your wants, needs and goals, and decide for yourself what type of life you want. As this is likely to be a new skill for you, consider hiring a coach to help you identify these things and build your confidence in staying true to your authentic self.

Part of your self-discovery will involve observing others—leaders, mentors, peers, staff—and trying to pinpoint what qualities you admire or loathe. Commit to spending a portion of your work-week networking because establishing yourself in your role and field is a lot about networking. Yes, the dreaded "n" word. Many of us dislike networking because it feels artificial and self-serving at best, completely transactional at worst. But what if it doesn't have to be like that? What if you transform your mindset to view networking as a mutually beneficial and even pleasurable activity?

If you are willing to suspend your judgment for a moment, here is a mindset about networking that you can adopt: networking helps other people meet their goals. That's right—it is not all about you, it's about them. Within your institution, you are part of a system. We all know this to some extent, and often do not consider the interplay of factors that comprise the system, how interdependent we all are. You were hired with a set of expectations that your department chair or division director is counting on you to achieve because, in aggregate, combined with the expectations of all your colleagues, that is how your boss's performance is measured by the Dean, whose performance is measured in turn, by the collective achievements of all faculty members in the college and trustees.

You can also think about networking at the level of your lab, clinic, or classroom. Every leader is measured on the achievements of those who work with them. Therefore, we are all invested in one another's success. Networking allows us to help others, which helps us and vice versa.

Before we address the how of networking, let's start with the *who*. First, there's you and you having done the work of knowing who *you* are. Now, the job is to understand yourself in relation to *others*. Start with organizational ("org") charts. Even within one institution, you can be part of multiple systems, including the college, university, hospital, residency program, research institute, cancer center, ambulatory center, etc. What is the relationship between these systems? Who is at the head of each one? How do they work together? What do they do? Who signed your letter of offer, contributes to your performance review or otherwise assigns you work? These are your primary stakeholders.

If you have not been given an onboarding plan, create your own. An onboarding plan is a standardized process that introduces you to the organization and helps you get to know the system and the interrelationship between its parts. Through onboarding you will learn about the systems you have access to and how they are used, the basic requirements of your job, and your team members and leaders. Starting with your roles, meet with the leader of each of your functional units. For instance, if you are a clinical faculty member in an outpatient clinic, you also teach in the residency program, and conduct quality-based research, consider meeting with your division director, department chair, medical director of the outpatient site, residency program director, departmental chair for quality, and chair of faculty development within the first 6 months of your appointment. You are seeking to learn what they do and how you can contribute to their successes. Within the first year, also meet with their bosses—the relevant associate and vice deans and Dean and hospital leaders and administrators. Note that it is a best practice to meet with those nearest to you in the org chart before venturing higher up. This is true of networking and definitely with respect to conflict resolution (see Chap. 9).

As for the *how*, just email. You can also stop by their office or call. But email is most common, and if these individuals have administrators, copying them on the email will likely yield a quicker response. What do you say in the email? Here's a template:

> "Dear Dr. ___,
>   As you may know, I am a new faculty member in ___ and as part of my onboarding, I would appreciate a meeting with you to learn more about ___. Would you be available for a half hour meeting within the next month?"

It's that simple. During the meeting, ask them about their role, their area, how they function within the bigger system, and tell them a bit about who you are—your area of expertise and goals. If there is something you hear that interests you or you want to contribute to—say so. Or directly ask for opportunities and recommendations. You should also ask for recommendations or introductions to potential collaborators, mentors, or other more senior leaders. It is a rare leader who ignores the interested. And if you reach out and don't get a response within a couple weeks, follow-up. It is easy to believe that they are too busy for you or disinterested, and that is rarely the case. Instead of making up a story or worrying about being a "bother," follow-up. I once worked with a leader who only responded to a third email (note that we do not endorse this tactic).

And one quick side note—always, and we do mean always, treat administrative staff with respect and kindness. There are two reasons for this. One, all people deserve respect, and two, administrators are an amazing source of information. If you want to know what is *really* going on in your institution, just ask an admin.

Your peers are another valuable source of information and connection, and in fact, can also be mentors. A peer who is only a year or two ahead of you is an incredibly valuable source of knowledge and perhaps easier to relate to than more senior mentors who are further from what you're currently experiencing. Cultivating relationships with peers across disciplines can be a source of support that augments your professional growth and provides a sense of connection and belonging within the organization.

You might find these peers within the same building in which you practice, research or teach. Have lunch or coffee in a common space, sit down with someone you don't know, or strike up a conversation in the elevator. I can hear the introverts groaning, and yet, as an introvert myself, I (Heather) can assure you that it is not that scary. Just ask, "what do you do?"

However, if you would prefer a more structured approach to meeting peers, try your faculty development office. Your college likely has an office and one or more deans dedicated to faculty development. They host workshops and webinars that are designed to teach you exactly what you need to know to be successful, and provides a great way to connect with colleagues. While any workshop provides an opportunity to connect, cohort programs will provide more in-depth touch points and even greater opportunities for sustained relationship-building.

A question we are often asked is, how do I find a mentor? First, do your research. What is it that you are interested in knowing or learning? Once you know what you want, you find a mentor by simply asking! Neither of us has ever met a person who spent a career in academia and was unwilling to mentor an early-career colleague. Don't let someone's seniority hold you back from reaching out to express interest in their work or to seek advice. And remember, just because a faculty member has seniority or a leadership role, doesn't necessarily make a person a good mentor! A colleague of mine (Kim), Dr. David Yousem, MD, MBA, has two great slides that we use in our mentoring talks. He phenotypes bad mentors as: dementors; lamentors; fomenters; tormentors; cementors; and fermenters. His phenotype of good mentors are: augmentors; implementors; supplementors; experimentors; commentors; and documentors.

So, find the good mentors and also be a good mentee (and a good mentor when your time comes). Good menteeship involves: setting regular appointments and showing-up on-time and ending on-time (or early); communicating clearly about your goals and needs; sending agenda emails and follow-up thank-you emails; respecting your mentors by demonstrating that you've done or explored what they recommended you do; and finally—showing gratitude to them! Note that you are not beholden to do whatever your mentors suggest—in fact, sometimes all the advice you get will conflict. You can then fall back on your grounding—who you are and what matters to you—trust yourself.

Know that a good mentor doesn't have to be the exact person you want to become; in fact, we strongly recommend having a team of mentors that can guide you through the many domains of your life and career [1]. We promote building a team of mentors because no one person can be your go-to for all the heterogeneous dimensions of your career and life [2]. We should all have career mentors, process mentors, promotion mentors, work-life integration mentors, peer mentors, etc.! [3].

Ultimately, what is behind this networking and relationship-building is the opportunity to gain multiple perspectives about the organization to usher your success. Networking helps you understand a culture's priorities and where your talents can best be applied. And let's not sugarcoat it, what you learn is also crucial for navigating organizational politics. Politics are embedded in the social structure of the organization; it's what motivates people and explains how employees use power and influence to foster personal agendas. You may be thinking that you have no interest in office politics and want to stay out it; unfortunately, this is not possible. However, you can lessen the pain of politics by understanding what is at play and who the players are. The org charts that you so diligently studied and the leaders that you have met through your onboarding process have what is called *positional authority*, stemming from their titles and where their roles reside in the organization. Their level of influence, however, may be equal to, lesser than, or greater than their titles. Similarly, you will meet people who have little positional authority and wield significant influence via *relational authority*. They are the people who know how to get things done, who have a finger on the pulse of the organization.

Knowing these people will help when you encounter an inevitable roadblock keeping you from doing what you were hired to do. It could be small—like getting a piece of equipment ordered—or it may be large—like encountering resistance to opening a new clinic in your specialty practice area. After a couple attempts of emailing or speaking to the person you believe to be in charge and getting nowhere, you will have to enter the political ring.

This entails using your network to understand the dynamics at play. Much like networking, this process is best undertaken by working your way up the chain of command, always starting with the person who is both nearest to you and to the decision-making. For instance, that might be the procurement department manager or your department administrator, for ordering equipment, your division director, department chair, or relevant medical director when it comes to opening the clinic.

"Help me understand," you might say, *"what can be done to get this accomplished?"* Notice the phrasing—you are demonstrating curiosity, you are not blaming the other person, and you are inviting them into the problem-solving process. You will also gather intel from your peers about whether they too have encountered similar situations and how they have handled them. With your mentors, you may ask them what they know and who might be able to help solve the issue.

What you are likely to discover is that through no fault of your own, or anyone else's really, your agenda is perceived to be in conflict with someone else's. A colleague thinks she has dibs on the space where your new piece of equipment is supposed to be housed, and she has the ear of the person who approves expenditures, consequently it has not been ordered. Or another group thinks that the clinic you are supposed to open will divert their patients and thus their revenue, and they have the ear of the Chief Medical Officer (CMO) who has not yet shared this information with your chair, and so on. And although this isn't your problem, it becomes your responsibility to broker a solution so that you can do your job. This is politics.

As you seek to accomplish your goals, two things will be particularly helpful to you, one is positioning your agenda in the interest of the organization and the other is listening to the concerns of others so that you can effectively influence the decision makers. Note that you are not solving the problem, per se, you are seeking out useful information and feeding it to the decision makers so that they can assuage concerns and jostle things around. You're like an expediter. For instance, perhaps your research mentor tells you that there is an unoccupied corner of someone else's lab, and that person may also benefit from this piece of equipment. That bit of information facilitates the solution, but it is not your direct responsibility to make it happen. It allows the research center director to talk to the person, gain assurance, and thus be the hero in making three people happy with this solution. With the clinic, perhaps a peer tells you that she heard your department administrator give a presentation about expanding the referral base for your specialty. A check-in reveals that the models have been run and they anticipate that your new clinic will be populated almost entirely by a new referral base that is being cultivated. This information is useful for the department chair who can then articulate an expansion plan to the CMO that satisfies the concerns of the other group, and again, facilitates a win for all parties. It's not always this easy, of course, and you can see how assumptions may cause intentions to become misconstrued. By being the person who commits to the best interest of the organization as a whole, even though you may be entering the political fray, you will not succumb to it and will build a reputation as a person who is fair and equitable.

And it is worth saying, when it comes to organizational politics, pick your battles wisely. The above examples illustrate barriers that directly impede your ability to carry out your agenda - without which, you won't have a job. Be wary of the issues that might affect your ability to do your job, and also affect a lot of other people. These are leadership's responsibility to address. A client of mine (Heather) once took on parking at her institution. Yes, access to parking affected her, though this was a universal challenge. She spent countless hours in meetings about parking and despite being justifiably outraged and able to convey that message on behalf of her peers, she had little influence and even less ability to effect change. This was not her battle.

It takes about a year to begin to feel comfortable in a new role, and perhaps even longer when that new role is also in a new place. Allow yourself the space and grace to be uncomfortable and unsure of yourself. Quite simply—you don't know what you don't know, and this period will allow you to learn so that when you do start to make your mark, you will be able to do so without wasting energy. This is a great time to refer to Chap. 3—"Who Are You?" because everyone is going to tell you to establish a niche.

A niche is your unique value proposition, the special thing that you bring to the table. It is often a skill, method, technique or area of inquiry that you pursue and to which you apply high quality contributions in one of the academic mission areas or aims (see Chap. 1). It may be the thing you were hired to do, for instance if you are a clinical sub-specialist, you already have a niche, ditto if you are a researcher. If you are a generalist, a hospital-based practitioner or an educator, your niche likely requires more effort on your part to be carved out. However, a subspecialist may want to distinguish themselves as an educator and may choose to develop a career focus as an expert in resident education, which only draws in part on their clinical expertise.

At this stage I hope you are asking, "how does one develop their niche and why does it matter?" First, the *why*. As was discussed in the first chapters, academia exists to disseminate knowledge. And this is the basis of the academic reward system—promotion in rank. Your job therefore is to distinguish your expertise and become a "go-to" to advance the body of knowledge within your field.

The harder part is *how*. This is where all the pieces begin to come together. Let's go back to the offer that you negotiated. Your letter sets the terms of your appointment with respect to how your time is allocated. If you are 90% clinical and 10% research and want to distinguish yourself as a bench scientist, that is not likely going to be feasible because 10% is not enough time for the lab. This is why it is important to be incredibly clear from the start about your objectives. However, with 10% protected time, you could do other forms of scholarship, including writing and publishing case studies, implementing industry-initiated clinical trials, perhaps developing an investigator-initiated trial, conducting quality studies, publishing how-to's about your techniques, getting involved in national committees or with advocacy and public policy efforts, etc. When these activities are aligned with your clinical practice, the output won't feel like too much "extra" work, so you can choose a method of scholarship that interests you.

If you are more of a generalist, you can find a niche within a broad scope of practice by observing what is missing in the current environment. Fortunately, you had a thorough onboarding and are a prodigious networker, so you already have some sense of what the needs are, and what else do you hear your colleagues discussing? What do people complain about? Where do the gaps seem to be? If you are an adult psychiatrist and hear your colleagues describe frustration with how ED consults are done, perhaps this is a problem you'd like to tackle? If taken on in a scholarly manner, the outcomes can be disseminated and even published and you will be the "go-to" person for improving ED psych consults, both within your home institution and for other hospitals. You can parlay this expertise into a national reputation as discussed in Chap. 7.

Distinguishing yourself as an educator often begins in your home department. Clinical departments will have residency and fellowship program directors that can help you learn about opportunities, as can associate deans or anyone who is actively engaged with teaching. While historically, many faculty members have "fallen into" teaching as a career focus, it is becoming more common for those interested in education to receive training in teaching techniques, methodology and assessment, as well as to further the science of education through research and scholarship [4, 5].

No matter what you choose, as you begin your career, save everything! Label email folders to help you save things such as: requests to lecture, invitations to present, thank you's or "kudos" from patients or colleagues, requests to review manuscripts, clinical usage reports, quality metrics, etc. This information will come in handy in the future when you write your promotion dossier. And speaking of promotion, early in your appointment, it is important to read your department's appointments, promotion and tenure document. This will help you understand by what you are going to be measured so that you can be intentional about what you do.

Practically speaking, there are several other things to pay attention to in the first years of an appointment. The first is *burnout*, which has a high degree of occurrence in early career and early in new leadership roles. Early burnout stems in part from overwork and trying to do too many things for too many people [6]. This is why you created a mission statement. It helps you decide what to say yes and no to. Also manage expectations, both your own and what others can expect of you. Regarding your own expectations—it is not possible to do everything all at once. Consider making a 5-year plan by working backwards from a longer-term goal and dividing that up into annual goals, and from there bi-annual goals. This will help you stay focused on what is feasible in a year and reduce the sense of overwhelm that can come from big aspirations.

Similarly, as you launch, be mindful how you are *'showing-up'*; that is, what precedent are you setting? Think of it this way, if after 3 years of coming in every day at 6 am and leaving every night at 6 pm, you start coming in at 7 am and leaving at 5 pm, those around you are going to perceive that you are slacking off, while the opposite would be perceived as extra dedication. So, while it is not impossible to establish a new precedent, it is significantly easier to add than remove (note: we do not endorse 12-hour workdays and studies demonstrate that productivity decreases as work hours increase).

Points to Ponder
- Who has positional authority in my organization, especially related to my areas of work?
- What do I find comfortable or uncomfortable about networking? How can I overcome any barriers or negative attitudes that I might have about it?
- What do I want to have done or achieved in 5 years—not just in my career but in the whole of my life?

- What is the unique skill, method, technique, knowledge or expertise that I bring? How can I leverage this relative to organizational gaps to create a niche?

Notes

References

1. Binkley PF, Brod HC. Mentorship in an academic medical center. Am J Med. 2013;126(11):1022–5.
2. Murrell AJ. Five key steps for effective mentoring relationships. Kaitz Quart. 2007;1(1):1–9.
3. Skarupski KA, Haythornthwaite J. Faculty longitudinal career mentoring. Invited chapter. In: Mentoring in health professions education: evidence-informed strategies across the continuum. IAMSE manuals. Cham: Springer; 2021.
4. Bartle E, Thistlethwaite J. Becoming a medical educator: motivation, socialisation and navigation. BMC Med Educ. 2014;14:110. https://doi.org/10.1186/1472-6920-14-110.
5. Mashauri HL. Who should be a medical educator? Beyond knowledge and experience. Ann Med Surg (Lond). 2023;85(10):4650–2. https://doi.org/10.1097/MS9.0000000000001200.
6. Dyrbye LN, et al. Burnout among US medical students, residents, and early career physicians relative to the general US population. Acad Med. 2014;89(3):443–51.

Chapter 6
Minding the "Academic" in Medicine

The first 6 months of your job will be spent onboarding, which can be exhausting. There are many bureaucratic hurdles you must jump to become "official" in your new role. Some of those tasks begin even before you move to your new institution. Credentialing, certifications, hospital privileges, health screening, federally-mandated learning modules, and the like are just some of the items that must be documented. Once you arrive, you will likely be invited to attend a new faculty orientation where you'll meet the school leaders and learn about policies and procedures, professionalism, promotion, and resources to support your career development.

After you've found the restrooms, figured-out who are the key administrative staff members, where to park, how to maneuver in the electronic medical record, and how to work with your institutions' office of research administration and institutional review board process, you'll want to establish a good habit of writing.

In academia, scholarship is the currency of the trade. If you're a faculty member, writing is an important part of your job, so do your job every day! Don't panic—that doesn't mean that you should be writing for 4 hours each day. If you have a clinical practice, even 10 minutes a day will move your research and papers along. My (Kim) colleague and friend, David Yousem, MD, MBA, is a neuroradiologist at Hopkins and advocate of faculty development. In a session we developed titled, "Get that paper out the door!" Dave always gives this example: the average article in the American Journal of Neuroradiology is 17 paragraphs long. If you write just one paragraph a week, after 52 weeks (one calendar year), you will have written three manuscripts. One paragraph a week! So after 7 years at the same rate, you will have written 21 manuscripts, which roughly corresponds to the publication benchmark most institutions require for promotion. Imagine if you wrote 2–3 paragraphs a week?

One tool to help you establish a sustainable writing habit is to start or join a writing accountability group (WAG). I (Kim) started WAGs (wagyourwork.com) at

Hopkins in 2013 based on an idea my former mentee, Kharma Foucher, MD, PhD, came up with when we were both at Rush University Medical Center. Several hundreds of WAGs, dozens of national presentations, a manuscript, workbook, a website, recorded learning modules, and ancillary tools have resulted; all to help you establish a sustainable habit of writing. I credit Paul Silvia's work (How to Write a Lot, and Write it Up) for describing the writing *process* and WAGs provide you with a writing *structure*.

WAGs are active writing groups comprised of 4–8 people who meet hourly, once a week for 10 weeks. A WAG follows a strict agenda of 15 min of updates and goal-setting followed by 30 min of individual writing, and then 15 min of reporting and wrap-up. Participants report: increased writing productivity (quantity and quality); greater control over the writing process; improved goal-setting and time-management skills; and as a bonus, an enriched sense of community.

WAGs work because they embed writing (and accountability) into your weekly calendar. Calendar appointments keep us accountable. Unless pressed with emergencies or urgencies, most of us strive to make our appointments. Making an appointment with yourself to write, think, network, read, etc. induces the same responsibility. Organization, combined with a commitment to our priorities, is key to good time management [1].

Time management is absolutely critical if you wish to have a successful career in academic medicine; otherwise, you will find yourself utterly consumed with the daily *urgent and important* facets of your life. Recall the Eisenhower Matrix we first presented in the Introduction (google it to see the graphic). Also known as the Stephen Covey or Urgent-Important Matrix, this is a productivity tool that helps prioritize tasks based on their urgency and importance. It categorizes tasks into four quadrants: important and urgent, important but not urgent, urgent but not important, and neither urgent nor important, aiding you in allocating time and effort effectively [2].

These urgent and important things, referred to by Stephen Covey as being within the quadrant of necessity, are your patient and clinic responsibilities, the critical logistics of running your research program(s), and the basics of managing your home and family. The problem is that many of us spend way too much time in the quadrant of urgent and not important, appropriately called the quadrant of deception by Covey. We deceive ourselves into believing these things are more important than they really are. But look at the types of tasks that end up in this quadrant—meetings, emails, non-life-or-death problems, some reports or compliance clicks. They are typically tasks and activities that demand immediate attention but don't contribute significantly to long-term goals or objectives. These tasks are often distractions or interruptions that can be delegated, minimized, or eliminated to focus on more meaningful and impactful activities. And note what else is similar about these items—they tend to be someone else's priority. Or worse, someone else has made their urgency your emergency.

This happens a lot in academic medicine because we are rewarded for our individual contributions. And, we know we're going to need help from others to advance our goals, so we try to play nice for mutual benefit. But sometimes this crosses a line and we need to address the situation and set boundaries. Establishing boundaries is essential to prevent one person's urgency from consistently overshadowing your responsibilities (I—Kim—frequently remind my coaching clients that 'we train people how to treat us'). Setting boundaries includes defining criteria for what constitutes genuine urgency and adhering to agreed-upon protocols for handling urgent requests. This also requires being mindful of tendencies to people-please and requires learning how to say no [3].

Learning to say no is important because if you don't actively schedule *your* time for *your* priorities, you will find that the tasks in the *not urgent but important* quadrant, also known as the quadrant of quality and personal leadership, the things like your career progress and scholarship, get neglected. To pay more attention to this facet, it is important to prioritize activities that contribute to long-term goals, personal growth, and strategic planning. Many items in this quadrant are proactive, preventative, or focused on improvement rather than immediate deadlines. In addition to putting time in your calendar, breaking down larger goals into smaller actionable steps, scheduling regular reviews of progress, and avoiding the temptation to constantly respond to urgent but less important tasks will help you stay focused on what really matters.

Other academic work that is not urgent yet important is participating in peer review. This involves reviewing manuscripts from academic journals within your field, critically evaluating them for scientific rigor, relevance, and clarity, and providing constructive feedback to authors. This process not only contributes to maintaining the quality and integrity of scholarly publications but also offers an invaluable opportunity for staying up-to-date on current research trends and methodologies. Naturally, by subscribing to the journals in your field and scheduling time to peruse the contents, you will stay abreast of the latest research findings, advancements, opinions, and clinical guidelines. Allocating dedicated time for journal reading and actively engaging with articles through critical analysis and reflection ensures continuous professional development and informs evidence-based practice in academic medicine.

This 'engagement' practice also extends to conferences. Conferences are essential for networking, learning, and sharing insights with peers from different institutions. They provide opportunities to stay abreast of the latest research, advancements, and best practices within your field. However, with so many conferences to choose from, and having a limited amount of time and professional development dollars, it's important to select the conferences that are best aligned with your professional goals and interests. Prioritize conferences that feature reputable speakers, relevant topics, and sessions that address current challenges and advancements in your area of expertise. Additionally, evaluating the conference's format, location, and opportunities for networking and collaboration can help determine whether to attend.

Building your research lab or program also requires teamwork. You'll need to find some good mentors—including administrators and peers—who can help you navigate your institutions' office of research administration, institutional review board, and other research-affiliated units. Your division or department may also have a vice chairperson of research who can help you navigate the research maze.

Don't be shy about asking your leaders and colleagues for copies of their recently funded grant applications. If you've never written a grant application before, seeing what a successful one looks like is pure gold! If you're exploring federal funding via the National Institutes of Health (NIH), you should bookmark their NIH RePORTER website that lists all funded grants. You can do a quick search by topic and the list pops-up and you can explore more details therein. You can also search by year, principal investigator, organization, and agency/institute/center. You can also explore the NIH's early career reviewer (ECR) program. Other large federal funding agencies common to academic medicine research include the Agency for Healthcare Research and Quality (AHRQ), the National Science Foundation (NSF), the U.S. Department of Defense (DOD), and the U.S. Department of Health and Human Services (HHS). Another good website is Grants.gov. They have a grant-writing basics blog series and a Grants Learning Center.

You might also want to explore non-traditional sources of funding for your research program. Build a relationship with your institution's office of development; meeting with them will provide an opportunity to share your research expertise and interests so that they might explore alignment with local benefactors and foundations, industry, grateful patients, and other potential funding sources and collaborators.

Finally, there is ongoing professional development. Clinicians are required to engage in CME (continuing medical education) and to earn CEUs (continuing education unit) and all faculty members are strongly urged to participate in ongoing professional and career growth, referred to as faculty development. Your school or institution likely has an office or center that specializes in offering a range of workshops, seminars, and mentoring opportunities designed to address the specific needs and challenges faced by faculty members. There are many skills that aren't taught in medical school, graduate school or residency, such as leadership and communication skills, many of which are addressed in these chapters.

I (Heather) created such an office at my former institution as a means for all faculty members to gain a full range of critical skills to support their professional goals. By actively participating in faculty development, faculty members also cultivate a supportive network of colleagues, gain valuable insights into academic administration, and ultimately learn how best to contribute to the overall excellence of medical education and research within their institution. Our data demonstrated that over a 10-year period, we were more likely to retain the faculty members who participated in our faculty development programming (89% retention) compared with their counterparts who did not participate (67% retention).

There are thousands of faculty members in academic medicine who have figured-out how to balance their: clinical, teaching, research, and life roles. You can too! Schedule your research time and guard it zealously. Start a WAG to hold you accountable to writing and to help you build a sustainable habit of writing. Invest in yourself and don't avoid the 'important, but not urgent' quadrant. Use your faculty annual review as a tool to set achievable goals and to celebrate your successes.

Points to Ponder
- If someone were to audit my calendar for a month, how would they depict a pie chart of where I spend my time?
- Where do I waste time? What time of day am I at my best?
- What tools can I use to prioritize my goals?
- What are my writing habits?
- What is one thing I can do immediately to prioritize my long-term goals?

Notes

_____
_____

References

1. Allen D. Getting things done: the art of stress-free productivity. Penguin; 2015.
2. Covey SR. The 7 habits of highly effective people. Simon & Schuster; 2020.
3. Tawwab NG. Set boundaries, find peace: a guide to reclaiming yourself. Westminster, London: Penguin; 2021.

Further Reading

Clear J. Atomic habits: an easy & proven way to build good habits & break bad ones. Penguin; 2018.

Chapter 7
Promotion

Promotion is the currency of trade in academic medicine—the 'coin of the realm.' It is the reward that distinguishes achievement in this environment from all others and signifies your expertise and experience. Promotion opens doors to leadership positions, both within your home institution and in national organizations. Promotion grants a legitimacy that is independent of the other skills you bring to the table. We have witnessed associate professors with marginal leadership skills get appointed to leadership positions over more highly-skilled assistant professors simply because of rank. Here's the thing—you are going to do the work anyway. You can either do a bunch of stuff and not get promoted or do a bunch of stuff and get promoted. While it may seem opaque or intimidating, if you follow the guidance here and share your intention with others, you'll get what you need and learn that it's not as hard as it seems.

For the individual, academic promotion in rank is an event that typically occurs just twice in the course of an entire career. For institutions, it is a regular process with rules and guidelines that make *War and Peace* look like a quick read. And yet, promotion is perhaps the most fraught topic in academic medicine. It is precisely this combination of rarity and rules that strikes fear in the hearts of many, with attrition being an unfortunate outcome of lack of understanding, particularly on the non-tenure tracks.

Therefore, the objective of this chapter is to demystify this topic with guidance that can be applied to any faculty member at any school, thus resulting in more faculty members being less daunted by the process and seeking the rewards they deserve.

Your eventual promotion is one of the key reasons to know the requirements of the different tracks and paths when you are being recruited. In this way, you can advocate for that which best suits your talents, skills, and interests. This is because the tracks and pathways have different sets of requirements and you want to maximize the work that is relevant to promotion and minimize that which is not [1, 2]. Importantly, however, is not to do things *only* for the sake of getting promoted. This strategy has a tendency to backfire.

We highly recommend having a plan for promotion based on your track and path. And reminder: these requirements should be aligned to the way in which your time is allocated. Therefore, if the way you spend your time changes, either out of necessity or due to your own interests shifting, you may find yourself on the "wrong" path and need to switch. Most institutions allow this, and our best guidance here is to not wait until you are ready for promotion, but to be proactive from the moment that your time has shifted.

Each promotion track and path has a set of criteria that a candidate must meet to be considered for promotion. The evaluation criteria encompass scholarship, teaching, and service domains. Depending on the emphasis within your career, one of these facets will hold greater significance and serve as the primary focus during your promotion review. However, activity in all areas is likely to be required. There are often quantifiable metrics for promotion, such as the number of publications a candidate is required to produce, or the number and variety of teaching materials a candidate is to have developed. Your plan for promotion begins with backtracking from these quantifiable metrics to give you a target of products to produce each year. Seek clarity!

Here's an example. Your department's Appointments, Promotion and Tenure document states that extramural funding is required for your track and path. Your department-level promotion committee chair tells you that means you need to have NIH funding. Your dossier is also reviewed by a separate college committee. The chair of that committee tells you that any form of extramural funding "counts" for promotion, it doesn't have to be NIH funding. How do you find out who's right? For starters, it's going to require a bit of diplomacy, and you may find having to navigate this situation annoying. That's understandable, so try to keep your attention focused on what is important, which is the clarification you need now to preclude problems later. Presuming that the department has the first say in whether you can proceed with promotion, that's the place to start. Go back to the departmental promotion chair and share what you learned.

But wait, there's more! As you dive into your promotion document, you'll notice terms like "excellence" and "reputation" sprinkled throughout. Deciphering these words often leads to the bulk of confusion during the promotion journey. They could be deemed the "hidden" requirements, subtly embedded, yet crucial. Think of them as the "we know it when we see it" standards; they're not as straightforward to measure as publication counts and can vary based on each person's career path.

We cannot emphasize this enough—do not make assumptions about what 'excellence' or 'reputation' means and how you will demonstrate it. There are many people in your institution who can help you understand what these words mean in practical terms. For starters, find out who the person is in your unit who oversees promotion. Schedule a meeting with this person early in your appointment. Tell them about yourself and that you are planning for promotion. Ask them a few key questions including, how does the promotion process work here? How will I know that I've achieved the requirements? How will I know that my work demonstrates excellence? How can I document my national and international impact? How is reputation defined? Who are some people similar to me who have been promoted? What advice would you give me?

Based on your institution's unique promotion process, you may want to meet with other people as well (e.g., faculty members who serve on promotions committees). One aspect that is universally consistent is that promotion dossiers are reviewed by a group of your peers, typically those at senior rank. These may be colleagues you work with every day, people you have never met, or a combination. Your dossier may go through several levels of review, starting at the local level—the department—and progress up through college and/or university-level reviews. It's important to know who will read your dossier because that determines in part how to present your material. If it's only read by people who know you well, you can get away with acronyms and there is a shared understanding of what is important. But the further away from your discipline that this document gets, the less people are going to understand the significance of activities germane to your field, meaning the more effort you will have to put forth to explain it. Therefore, if your promotion goes through reviews at other levels, also meet with the people who oversee the reviews at those other levels. Ask them the same questions you ask at your local level. And expect different answers. This is where the notion of interpretation comes in. Your job is to calibrate the information you are getting by sharing any discrepancies and asking for clarification.

You should know that what constitutes "academic" work looks different in every institution. In Chap. 2, we touched on Boyer's classification of scholarship [3], which informs the promotion and tenure guidelines of many institutions, and yet the interpretation of what "counts" in each of the categories at each institution is often a matter of culture and preference. At large schools, this may even differ significantly between departments within the same college. Therefore, when considering the academic piece of academic medicine, it is wise to identify the norms of your environment. Points of contention are often about quantity vs quality, the type and quality of funding to sustain one's work, and how impact of scholarship is assessed.

A faculty member at my (Heather) former institution had a prolific publication record and was denied promotion because the vast majority of his scholarship was in non-peer reviewed open access journals, therefore it was not deemed to have sufficient quality. Another faculty member published exclusively in high impact journals and only had three publications at the time of promotion-review because she had emphasized perfection and extremely high quality over quantity. Thus, she suffered from having few citations to demonstrate the impact of her work. Yet another faculty member was denied promotion because she didn't have NIH funding, despite the fact that her research program was easily sustained and impactful without it. Yet another faculty member was turned down because his teaching evaluations were deemed to be too low; however, he also had the fewest number of evaluations as his teaching was primarily at a sister school, and those high evaluations were not considered in the department's overall assessment. These examples are not provided to scare you, but to demonstrate how better knowledge and guidance early on likely would have avoided these denials.

Your candidacy is also likely to be evaluated by peers from other institutions. This is known as the external review process. These peers usually cannot be current or former mentors, or people with whom you have collaborated or who otherwise stand to gain from your promotion. You may be asked to provide suggestions of credible people in your field, or you may not. You cannot try to influence the external review process while it's happening, though garnering name recognition in your field in advance of a promotion review is something that will serve you well. This is also known as building a reputation.

Becoming known in your field starts with your professional credibility. Meaning you produce high quality work and you do what you say you are going to do. All the networking in the world won't help you if you don't deliver. And this begins at the local level. Spend your first couple of years building your practice and demonstrating follow-through on your commitments to your patients, learners, and colleagues. This will make you a trusted colleague—one that others feel comfortable recommending. Being recommended by people who are already established in your field is a much easier path to developing a reputation than going it alone. However, it is up to you to guide others in recommending you for the right types of opportunities. This goes back to your mission and vision. The more clarity you have about where you want to go, the better you can help others help you get there. Which means that it also serves you well to know which of your colleagues are involved in the societies and organizations to which you may like to belong. When you know this, you can ask them for advice about how to get involved, to make introductions for you or to nominate you. Some mentors or department chairs will be proactive in this regard, others will not, and in our experience, this is merely a difference of style, it doesn't represent an unwillingness to support you—it just requires prompting on your part.

It is never wise to put all of your eggs in one basket; therefore, as you focus your attention on building credibility at home, it is also wise to begin to establish relationships with known experts in your field at the meetings and conferences you attend. Early-career faculty members often feel uncomfortable approaching a big name in the field; but trust us, everyone enjoys talking about their own work. Presenting a poster is another terrific way to engage in conversation, and for faculty who are less-oriented to traditional forms of scholarship, engaging in professional development programs offered in your specialty, taking part in a clinical task force, or otherwise volunteering to serve in a way that advances the profession and utilizes your unique skills and interests will help you get noticed.

As you progress in your academic career, you will want to have periodic check-ins to ensure that you are on track for promotion. If you are on the tenure track, you may have a finite amount of time before you will be required to go up for promotion, and within that time frame there is a thorough mid-point review to provide you with feedback about your progress. Faculty with a "clock" also have the opportunity to extend it for various reasons; typically inclusive of having a child, a sustained illness or period of caregiving for a family member, or an unexpected set-back that affected one's ability to conduct research.

For faculty without a mandate, the annual review meeting with the department chair or division director is a useful time to gauge progress toward promotion. Many faculty members, even associate professors, expect to be told that they are ready to go up for promotion, and yet, in our experience, that is not often the case. This is your career; therefore, you are in the driver's seat to express what it is you want and to seek the guidance and support you need to attain it. You'll likely find a willing network to support you, though with the pace of medicine today, this network is most likely to be responsive, not proactive, in helping you achieve your goals.

7 Promotion

So you've gotten promoted to associate professor—congratulations! Now what? This step can feel like a plateau, like the reward is getting to do more of the same for eternity. But it doesn't have to be! Getting promoted to associate professor gives you cache; it distinguishes you as a person who is a bona fide academic—a member of the club. And as a recent study demonstrated, only about 38% of assistant professors get promoted to associate professor, so this does indeed set you apart [4].

Once you get promoted to associate professor, you can expect to be invited to participate in more committees and service activities both within your institution and your profession. You can choose to be more selective about these requests, and use them to gain new skills and insights into how systems work. This is particularly helpful in a leadership journey, as discussed in the next chapter. Additionally, your assistant professor peers will regard you as a mentor and many people will seek your advice and guidance. There is visibility with the role, which can feel exhilarating, daunting and exhausting, sometimes all at the same time. All this while still building your own career.

It's no wonder that associate professors are more dissatisfied with their careers than their assistant professor and full professor colleagues [5]. This promotion can very much feel like the "reward" is more work. This career stage requires one to reevaluate priorities and goals, also because it tends to coincide with the time of life that faculty are also raising families and caring for aging parents. The overwhelm contributes to burnout, which prompts early departure from medicine or a change of institutions in hopes that the grass is greener [5, 6].

To begin the re-envisioning, think of the promotion to associate professor as a platform itself, not just a step in the rung on the ladder to professor. You are now in a position to more readily influence and shape your institution and profession. Reevaluate your values, mission and vision for your career. Consider how the context of your life has changed. Rather than being swept into the tidal wave of demands, consider how to make the prestige of your position work for you by setting boundaries and asking for what you need and want to support your continued growth. Assert your value. Revisit Chap. 3 ('Who am I? Why does it matter?') for guidance.

And this takes us to full professor. Advancing to the rank of full professor is a pinnacle achievement for many, and rightly so. Full professors are esteemed authorities in their respective fields, typically demonstrating a substantial body of scholarly work and widespread recognition at a national or international level. Attaining this rank requires notable contributions to professional service and a reputation as a respected leader in the field.

While the path to full professor mirrors that of associate professorship, the focus shifts towards amplifying existing accomplishments rather than establishing credibility anew. However, the fundamental strategies remain consistent. While there is limited literature on the transition from associate to full professor, the process largely involves similar metrics, albeit with heightened emphasis on demonstrable leadership and impact within the field. Mere participation is insufficient; institutions seek to elevate individuals who exhibit leadership qualities. Aspiring full professors should actively pursue leadership roles, engage in invited presentations, particularly as keynote speakers or guest lecturers, and aim to establish themselves as authorities in their specific areas of expertise, aligning with the increasingly specialized nature of modern medicine.

However, keep in mind that your career is a marathon, not a sprint. It will be very tempting to do all the things, which is a recipe for burnout and overwhelm. If you remain clear on *your* vision and mission, seek out guidance and support, and are consistent, you will set yourself up for success on your terms and benefit the profession, as well. This is what it means to do things for the right reasons.

Points to Ponder
- Who are the people in my institution that can help me understand the nuances of the promotion process?
- How am I letting others know what is important or meaningful to me so that they can help me?
- What is the impact that I want to have and how is impact defined by my institution?
- What makes my work important and how can I describe that?
- How does my institution describe reputation? How do I demonstrate mine?
- How will I reconcile conflicting information that I receive about promotion?

Notes

References

1. Roberts LW, editor. The academic medicine handbook: a guide to achievement and Fulfillment for academic faculty, Chapters 44–48. New York: Springer; 2013.
2. Mallon WT. The anatomy and physiology of medical school faculty career models. New Brunswick: Rutgers University Press; 2016. p. 81–100.
3. Boyer EL. Scholarship reconsidered: priorities of the professoriate; 1990. The Carnegie Foundation for the Advancement of Teaching.
4. Xierali IM, Nivet MA, Syed ZA, Shakil A, Schneider F, David MD. Recent trends in faculty promotion in U.S. medical schools: implications for recruitment, retention, and diversity and inclusion. Acad Med. 2021;96(10):1441–8.
5. Dyrbye LN, Varkey P, Boone SL, Satele DV, Sloan JA, Shanafelt TD. Physician satisfaction and burnout at different career stages. Mayo Clin Proc. 2013;88(12):1358–67.
6. Brod HC, Lemeshow S, Binkley PF. Determinants of faculty departure in an academic medical center: a time to event analysis. Am J Med. 2017;130(4):488–93.

Further Reading

Sanfey H, Hollands C. Career development resource: promotion to associate professor. Am J Surg. 2012;204(1):130–4. https://doi.org/10.1016/j.amjsurg.2012.04.004. https://www.sciencedirect.com/science/article/pii/S0002961012002139.

Chapter 8
Leadership

It seems that everyone wants to be a leader—of something. However, in academic medicine, leadership is a crucial aspect of any role you hold, whether it involves leading research or clinical teams, interacting with patients, families, and students, or collaborating with interdisciplinary and professional groups. Though you may not view yourself as a leader if you only view leadership through a *positional* lens. That is, if you think leaders are people like your: senior mentors; division and department leaders; famous clinicians, educators; scientists in your field; deans, and so forth, you may not think that *you* are a leader. But you are. You are already a leader! Look around you. If anyone is following you, admiring you, learning from you, or looking up to you—you're a leader.

Leadership extends far beyond formal titles. At its core, leadership is a set of behaviors. Yes, in any industry, leadership is likely based on some presumed technical expertise; but leadership is also the ability to communicate and negotiate effectively, make strategic decisions, diffuse conflict, inspire and motivate others, and navigate complex organizational dynamics. Positional leadership within an organization or society expands beyond leading teams to shaping the broader vision and strategy. It involves navigating complex organizational structures, fostering alignment across departments and disciplines, and advocating for resources and support to advance the institution's mission and values. Effective organizational leaders inspire confidence and trust through transparent communication, integrity, and a commitment to ethical decision-making. They prioritize diversity, equity, and inclusion, fostering a culture of belonging where all voices are heard and valued. Furthermore, organizational leaders cultivate partnerships and collaborations with external stakeholders, driving innovation, and enhancing the institution's reputation and impact on a global scale.

Leadership begins with the self. It starts with a deep understanding of one's own values, strengths, and areas for growth (see Chap. 3). Self-awareness is the cornerstone of effective leadership and is what enables people to show up authentically and lead with integrity. Leaders need the ability to see their own biases, know their emotions and limitations, and understand their cognitive compensation strategies. Additionally, self-leadership is about taking responsibility for your actions and decisions, even in the face of adversity or uncertainty. It involves cultivating resilience, perseverance, and a growth mindset to navigate challenges and inspire others to do the same.

Leading teams requires more than self-awareness; it necessitates an understanding of group dynamics and interpersonal relationships. Effective team leadership involves fostering a culture of trust, respect, and open communication, where each team member feels valued and empowered to contribute their unique perspectives and skills. A successful team leader identifies and leverages the strengths of each team member, while also providing guidance and support to address challenges and achieve common goals. Moreover, team leadership requires the ability to navigate conflicts constructively and to foster collaboration across diverse backgrounds and disciplines. Unfortunately, leading others is sometimes viewed merely as a rung on the career ladder, and this significant responsibility to others is overlooked. Therefore, if you aspire to lead others, it is critical to understand your motivations.

While some individuals may possess innate leadership qualities, leadership is primarily a learned skill. Seeking leadership training allows you to develop skills intentionally, enhancing the capacity to lead teams, drive innovation, and ultimately make a greater impact. By investing in leadership development, you can excel in your role and also contribute more effectively to the advancement of science and healthcare. Everyone can benefit from leadership development training, however, if you envision a career of formal leadership, it's vital to cultivate self-awareness, seek mentorship, and develop relevant skills such as communication and decision-making. To begin, actively pursue leadership development opportunities, demonstrate initiative through volunteering for leadership-related tasks, and build a strong professional network. Stay informed about industry trends and remain adaptable to new opportunities and challenges. By taking these steps, you can position yourself for success and advancement in leadership roles within academic medicine.

However, your first year may likely not be the right time to pursue formal leadership training because you'll be consumed with learning your job and the culture. Nevertheless, you can start to identify gaps in your professional development and pick one or two things to work on in your early-career. For instance, topics and skills that develop self-awareness are: emotional intelligence, personality preferences, and knowing your strengths. While discrete skills that will aid your growth include: being a better mentee; developing a sustainable writing practice and habit (see WAGs); improving your communication style; building a lab or clinical practice; managing and mediating conflict; and negotiating. You could identify one of these skills or some other one you'd like to develop and discuss it with your mentor(s) or department chair at your annual review. There are ample ways to learn and practice a new skill. A professional career development plan (PCDP) is a useful tool to help you and your mentors strategize your growth.

Most institutions offer leadership programs for faculty members. These leadership programs ordinarily are cohort-based and longitudinal, meeting on a set schedule over the course of months or a year. Additionally, many professional societies offer leadership programming, minimally offering leadership workshops in conjunction with annual conferences or via online, stand-alone programming.

Leadership program curricula vary; you can use the self/other/organizational model, such as the one I (Heather) implemented in the Center for FAME at Ohio State, to identify what skills will be most helpful for a faculty member to develop at what career stage. When it comes to content, be sure to review the program's agenda to check for alignment with your goals. For example, Johns Hopkins University espouses 12 leadership competencies: establishing relationships; developing talent; inspiring and motivating others; demonstrating emotional intelligence; acting with integrity; acting strategically; managing risk; navigating organizations; communicating effectively; promoting diversity and inclusion; setting a strategic vision; and holding self and others accountable.

There are also ample leadership resources available online for self-study. For example, Harvard Business Review (HBR) has an "HBR Must Reads" series on Leadership [1] and there are countless titles if you search for leadership in Amazon.com (see References & Further Readings at the end of this chapter for some of our favorites). There are also a number of podcasts focused on leadership. The *Faculty Factory* podcast and YouTube channel covers a wide range of leadership topics in academic medicine. The *Maxwell Leadership Executive Podcast* is founded on John C. Maxwell's leadership books as is Patrick Lencioni's *At the Table* podcast. Brené Brown has a *Dare to Lead* podcast and Laura Knights' *Black Women Leading* is another. *Executive Minds* features leaders from corporate America and is focused on business leadership, while Kemi Doll's *Your Unapologetic Career* podcast primarily focuses on self-leadership and one's influence in academic medicine. When pressed for time, you can get key points and synopses of influential leadership books on sources like Blinkist.

As you're preparing for a future leadership position, how do you get noticed? Many early-career faculty members are mistakenly under the impression that leadership nominations arise spontaneously or are offered to the most qualified person. This is rarely the case. Most people get nominated for something because they ask for it, and they usually draft their own nominating statement and provide it to the nominator to edit. If there is an opportunity or award that you would like to be nominated for, ask the best person you know to make this nomination on your behalf (the criteria of the nominator will be found in the issuing statement). Offer to draft the letter and don't be modest. This is also good practice for writing your eventual promotion narratives, and your promotion CV or dossier.

You will also get noticed via presenting your work at national and international conferences. You should join your scientific field's professional society(ies) and attend their annual conference or meeting. Ideally, you are submitting abstracts to present your work at your annual conferences via podium presentations (oral talk), panels, workshops, posters, etc. You'll definitely get noticed if you volunteer to *actively* serve on any your society's steering committees and workgroups. You're also noticed when you find yourself getting invited to give lectures or presentations at other institutions or organizations. Invited presentations are coveted because they signal a person's reputation. An invited presentation is typically one for which you haven't applied. That is, if you submit an abstract and that abstract is selected for a presentation, it is *not* invited. But that doesn't mean that you can't solicit an invitation to present. Some schools have exchange programs for early-career faculty, some early-career faculty members ask their mentors or department chair to arrange an invitation, others will reach out to colleagues they know well at other institutions and offer to make a presentation. When these offers are accepted, an invitation is extended and therefore, congrats!—you now have an invited presentation to put in your promotion dossier. You can also use meetings and conferences to let others know that you are happy to come to their campus to present and be sure to follow-up to reiterate the offer once you get back home. With countless hours of Grand Rounds and other meeting slots to fill each year, names of presenters are always welcome.

Once you are convinced of your desire for a formal (positional) leadership role, how do you get one? You can start planting seeds of your leadership interests during your annual review with your supervisor or anytime with your mentor(s), peers, and colleagues in your professional societies. Start paying closer attention to the current roles in your area—who is doing what? Notice if there are gaps or unaddressed needs in your environment; you may be able to create a leadership role based on emerging needs and interests. Keep your eyes and ears open to shifting priorities and people; network to learn where opportunities may be arising because of new programs being built and/or people moving to other positions.

As you're perusing job sites (internally, within your institution or externally, outside your institution), you may come across a posting for a formal leadership role that interests you. You should read the job description very carefully and do your research. Regardless if you're considering an internal or external job, ask yourself these same questions: Is the role mission-centric? Does it align with my values? How would the job affect my assets; that is, my income and my time (think about your home and social life)? With whom can I meet to discuss what they know about the job and if they think I'd be a good fit? How can I learn more about the expectations, challenges, metrics for success, politics, budget, resources, etc.? What will I have to stop doing if I were to transition to this new role? Talk with your peers, mentors, relevant staff (if internal), and family/friends about the opportunity. If it's an external job, you might have to do some more in-depth internet searching to learn more about the institution; the department/division; leadership; their mission, vision, and values; their budget; their relationship with the community, trustees, and other stakeholders; politics, etc. For an external job, you should still reach-out to your mentors, peers and/or colleagues to learn what they know about the other institution/employer and the role. Similarly, you may end-up being recruited for other positions at external institutions; the same rules apply (do your homework and ask yourself the same questions above). When a recruiter contacts you for a promising opportunity, consider working with a job coach to guide you through the letter-writing/application process, telephone calls, initial online (Zoom) interviewing, in-person interviewing, and negotiating phases.

Leadership is great but it's also important for you to be aware of good followership skills. Good followers facilitate good leaders, and vice versa. We're all followers because we are all subordinate to and answer to at least one someone. What is good followership? Good followership is constructive critical thinking and interacting with the group and leader [2]. Good followers don't simply obey leaders blindly or passively, or worse, maliciously. Good followers think deeply about issues and when they courageously challenge their leader, it's done with a high degree of emotional intelligence. Good followers avoid groupthink (i.e., when everyone in a group thinks about and does things the same way) and when they choose to challenge the status quo, they do so by gauging their unique circumstances and then offering constructive alternatives [3]. Unlike leadership, we don't know of any courses specifically on followership, although at Hopkins we weave the concept of followership into our leadership programs, citing the references at the end of this chapter.

Beyond titles or positions, true leadership is about inspiring and empowering others, fostering collaboration, and driving positive change. It's about making a meaningful impact in the lives of patients, colleagues, and the broader community. Good leaders prioritize integrity, empathy, and ethical decision-making, striving to create inclusive environments where everyone feels valued and supported. As you progress in your leadership journey, continually reflect on your values, seek feedback, and remain committed to personal and professional growth. Embodying these principles will help you excel in your role and also make a lasting difference in your field. Remember, "whatever you are, be a good one" (Abraham Lincoln).

Points to Ponder
- Who are some good leaders I admire? What is it about them that I admire?
- Who are some good followers I admire? What do I admire about their followership style?
- What are the traits of some bad leaders I've known?
- What are my natural strengths as a leader?
- What are some of my blind spots? How can I identify my blind spots?
- What skills do I want to work on?

Notes

References

1. Harvard Business Review (HBR). HBR's 10 must reads. On leadership. Boston: Harvard Business Review Press; 2011.
2. Gibbons A, Bryant D. Followership: the forgotten part of doctors' leadership. BMJ. 2012;345:e6715. https://www.bmj.com/content/345/bmj.e6715
3. Chaleff I. The courageous follower: Standing up to and for our leaders. 3rd ed. Oakland: Berrett-Koehler Publishers; 2009.

Further Readings

Covey SR. The 7 habits of highly effective people: powerful lessons in personal change. New York: Free Press; 1989.

Goldsmith M. What got you here won't get you there: how successful people become even more successful. Hachette: UK Hachette Books; 2007.

Kouzes JM, Posner BZ. The leadership challenge: how to make extraordinary things happen in organizations. 5th ed. San Francisco: Wiley; 2012.

Skarupski KA. Invited Chapter. AAMC GFA Guidebook. Managing career transitions and succession. Co-editors: Gibson J, Freeman E, Ripley B, Hill J, Brazeau C, Rowland M, Best B, Love J, Runge C. 2020. https://www.aamc.org/professional-development/affinity-groups/gfa/leadership-guide-faculty-affairs-professionals.

Wiseman L. Multipliers: how the best leaders make everyone smarter. New York: Harper Collins Publishers; 2017.

Chapter 9
What to Do When (Not if) Things Get Rough

This is the dose of reality chapter. Even if you do everything we promote in this book, you may experience setbacks or not get the result that you desire. This is normal and feels terrible, which is why we want to share some thoughts and guidance on uncomfortable topics, including burnout, self-sabotage, mid-career malaise, conflict, and bullying.

Whatever your role in academic medicine, there's a high likelihood that you will experience burnout at some point in your career. According to an American Medical Association publication, at least 63% of practicing physicians experience symptoms of burnout once per week [1]. Burnout is characterized by emotional exhaustion, depersonalization, and a diminished sense of personal accomplishment. It often stems from the demanding nature of academic roles, including heavy workloads, high-pressure environments, and the expectation to excel in research, teaching and clinical duties, combined with systemic factors such as electronic medical records, administrative tasks and inequitable workload distribution.

It's essential to address burnout to ensure a lasting career in academic medicine. Since burnout often arises from systemic issues that diminish your sense of control, reclaiming your locus of control is a crucial initial step to combat burnout. A coach can assist you in recognizing your responses to various situations and identifying areas where you can exert influence to enact positive changes. Additionally, you can cope with burnout by prioritizing self-care, including setting boundaries, practicing stress-relief methods like mindfulness or exercise, seeking support from colleagues or mentors, and taking regular breaks to recharge. These measures do not cure the causes of burnout, but they are a salve for managing its effects.

Aside from burnout, you may experience career challenges stemming from many other factors, including circumstances in your personal life, or professional setbacks like not getting promoted or appointed to a leadership position. Your funding might run out, or your contract may not get renewed. In these circumstances, the question to ask yourself is—Did I put forth my best effort? If the answer is yes, then you can know that the situation was beyond your locus of control. This doesn't make the disappointment go away, but it can help you not internalize the setback and blame yourself. You can find your resolve to try again, or reach for a goal that better aligns with your strengths.

However, if you don't think you put forth your best effort, then you have arrived at a learning opportunity. First ask yourself, what prevented you from doing your best? Was it something internal or external? Meaning, did you do it to yourself or is it the result of things being done to you? Maybe it's a combination of both.

Things we do to ourselves include procrastination, perfectionism, imposter syndrome, not being appropriately assertive, overcommitting, not setting boundaries, failure to adapt, negative self-talk, poor time management, isolationism, not seeking or receiving feedback or help, ignoring health and well-being, comparison to others, as well as many other self-sabotage strategies, as described in a Chronicle of Higher Education article [2]. Throughout this book we have described tactics that will help you avoid these tendencies. However, you are human, and therefore, imperfect.

If you suspect that you have sabotaged yourself, reflection and an honest assessment of your behaviors and outcomes can be a learning opportunity to continue to develop self-awareness and grow into a better version of yourself. A few ways to do this are:

- *Reflection*: take some time to reflect on recent professional situations, decisions, and outcomes. Consider whether any patterns of behavior or choices may have contributed to negative outcomes.
- *Seek feedback*: Reach out to trusted colleagues, mentors, or supervisors and ask for honest feedback about your performance and behaviors. They may provide insights into areas where you might be inadvertently hindering your progress.
- *Examine Thought Patterns*: Pay attention to your thoughts and self-talk. Are you constantly doubting your abilities, fearing failure, or dismissing your accomplishments? These thought patterns can reveal self-sabotaging tendencies.
- *Evaluate Opportunities Taken or Missed*: Think about opportunities you've pursued or passed up. If you consistently avoid taking on challenges or shy away from new experiences, you might be holding yourself back.
- *Assess Relationships*: Consider how you interact with colleagues, supervisors, and subordinates. Are there any communication or relationship dynamics that might be impacting your professional growth?
- *Analyze Stress Levels*: Excessive stress, burnout, or consistently feeling overwhelmed can indicate that you might be engaging in behaviors that are detrimental to your well-being and performance.
- *Seek Professional Help*: If you're struggling to identify self-sabotaging behaviors on your own, consider seeking help from a career coach, therapist, or counselor. They can provide an external perspective and guide you toward self-improvement.

Another common phenomenon is when you find yourself wondering—*is this it*? Ironically, this thought tends to creep up when some sort of milestone has been reached—like a promotion, new leadership position, or significant birthday. It reveals that we had expectations about how we thought we *should* feel at this time, and reality isn't matching expectations [3]. Although this can happen at any point in our lives, it frequently occurs around mid-life, hence, the *mid-career malaise* [4]. If this is the spot you're in, the guidance provided in Chap. 3 (Who Am I? Why Does It Matter?) is worth revisiting. Sometimes we don't realize that we are wedded to a plan that is no longer serving us and it's time for a refresh.

When roadblocks in our academic careers are self-imposed, we wield considerable choice in overcoming them, often with the guidance of a coach. However, sometimes our challenges are external to us and cause a great deal of distress and shame. Things that others do to us include: harassment—sexual and otherwise; bullying; backstabbing; discrimination; predatory mentoring; toxic leadership; dishonesty or manipulation; violating ethical guidelines; and gaslighting (see the Appendix at the end of this chapter for descriptions of these behaviors). While many in academic medicine are not inclined towards such behaviors, encountering individuals who exhibit them can significantly derail your career. From my (Heather) experience coaching women in academic medicine, it's clear that when organizations fail to address such misconduct, it leads to trauma, stress, overwhelm, PTSD, and burnout among others. Unfortunately, this pervasive issue persists for reasons too numerous to detail here.

Nevertheless, akin to addressing the systemic nature of burnout, there are avenues to address abusive behavior in the workplace. Firstly, pinpoint the specific actions of the individual—the behaviors themselves, not just your interpretation or reaction to them. For example, "S/he was rude to me" is your perception vs. "S/he raised his voice, narrowed his/her eyes and said to me, 'who do you think you are'?" is a description of the behavior. Document these experiences, preferably using your work email. Simply send yourself an email detailing the incident for time-stamped and discoverable evidence in case of a formal complaint or legal action in the future.

Confronting the individual directly is a potential first step (except in cases of sexual harassment), albeit with caution regarding your safety. Opt for a conversation in a busy office or via telephone, possibly inviting a neutral observer or recording the conversation, particularly if retaliation or gaslighting is a concern. While confronting the person directly demonstrates assertiveness and may lead to resolution, it could also trigger defensiveness, escalation, or emotional tolls. Carefully choose your words, employing the 4-part communication strategy from *Nonviolent Communication* to keep the conversation non-confrontational and anticipate various outcomes (i.e., what I observe and what you observe; how I feel and how you feel; what I need or value and what you need or value; and the corrective actions I would like taken and the corrective actions you would like taken) [5, 6]. You can also learn more about your (and your colleagues') conflict styles (competing, collaborating, compromising, avoiding, accommodating) by taking the online Thomas-Kilmann conflict mode instrument assessment [7].

However, direct confrontation may not offer a lasting solution, especially in cases of persistent bullying, which may necessitate involvement from HR and management. Additionally, the hierarchical nature of medicine creates complex power dynamics that threaten a complainant's reputation and credibility, perpetuating a fear of retaliation and a reluctance of bystanders to come forward. If direct confrontation feels untenable or fails to resolve the situation, informal and formal channels within the organization can offer assistance. Initiate discussions with your supervisor or escalate to higher-level management, such as the dean or appropriate health system leaders, if necessary [8].

In matters concerning diversity, inclusion, or bias, you can address the issue with your institution's Office of Institutional Equity (OIE), which initiates investigations known as grievances. Institutional leaders are mandated reporters to the OIE, obligated to file a grievance on your behalf if you raise discrimination concerns with them. Your Human Resources office, Office of Faculty Affairs, and Title IX office also handle formal grievances related to interpersonal disputes, and offer guidance regarding procedures and potential outcomes. For complaints about research misconduct, patient safety, or student-related concerns, respective designated offices manage these issues with specialized procedures. Some organizations provide an ombudsman or mediation program for confidential discussions and impartial resolutions.

If your concern remains unresolved and poses significant risks to university reputation or personal safety, consider escalating it to campus authorities like campus police, provost, vice provost, or university president. Factor in the seriousness of the situation, relationships involved, and organizational protocols when deciding the escalation pathway. Maintain detailed records of interactions throughout the process, and approach it professionally with the aim of achieving a resolution beneficial to all parties. It's important to acknowledge that institutional leaders prioritize protecting the institution, which can create challenges in navigating difficult situations, often leaving individuals feeling marginalized and disregarded.

In such instances, seeking external legal counsel may be necessary. If disputes persist despite proper channels, involve retaliation, discrimination, or potential legal repercussions, consulting an attorney outside the institution can be advantageous. Legal guidance is particularly beneficial if the situation carries the potential for retaliation, reputational harm, or involves complex employment law issues. During an initial consultation, discuss your circumstances, goals, and any relevant documentation. This enables the attorney to provide personalized advice on potential legal options.

Through my (Heather) coaching experience, I've observed the tolerance of dysfunction and toxicity in academic medicine, often due to the perceived cost of addressing it. Consequently, faculty members endure silently, grappling with trauma, embarrassment, or shame. Let me be unequivocal—enduring disrespectful or dehumanizing treatment, boundary violations, or ethical compromises is never acceptable. Unfortunately, coming forward entails risks; therefore, it's important to assess the risks and potential consequences of your actions to make an informed decision that meets your needs.

When you encounter challenges or professional setbacks, there are resources available to support you, including coaches, therapists, and your institution's

Employee Assistance Program, all of which offer safe and confidential help. Peers and peer groups can provide a supportive community, while options like FMLA and sabbatical can offer leave from work to prioritize your health. And if necessary, there's no shame in seeking a new position, institution, or career that better aligns with your values and needs. Your well-being is paramount. Enduring harmful behavior can gradually erode your self-worth, making it incredibly challenging to address. If you sense something isn't right, trust your instincts and reach out to a trusted individual for support and guidance. You deserve to be treated with respect and dignity, and when you feel disempowered, appropriately advocating for yourself is a crucial step towards reclaiming your agency.

Points to Ponder
- How will I know if I'm getting burned-out? What behaviors will I exhibit?
- Do I engage in any self-sabotaging behaviors? What are they and what can I do about them?
- When was the last time I was in conflict? What is my conflict style? What was my contribution to the problem? What was imposed upon me?
- Do I recognize any of the bullying behaviors in myself or others? How can I advocate for myself and others?
- How can I make the nonviolent communication strategies a habit for when conflict arises?

Appendix: Types of Abusive Behaviors

Fortunately, these are not very common behaviors in academic medicine, and hopefully you will not come across them. However, as we are not taught about ways in which we cause harm to one another, we often don't have the language to articulate what we are experiencing. Below are some examples of common types of harmful behaviors.

Harassment or Bullying
- Verbal abuse, insults, derogatory language.
- Repeatedly singling out an individual for criticism or humiliation.
- Threats or intimidation, either in person or online.
- Isolation of the target from colleagues or social groups.
- Unwarranted interference with someone's work or personal space.

Backstabbing
- Spreading malicious rumors or gossip about someone.
- Taking credit for another person's work or ideas.
- Undermining a colleague's efforts or reputation behind their back.
- Betrayal of trust by sharing confidential information in a harmful way.

Predatory Mentoring
- Offering mentorship with hidden agendas, such as seeking personal gain or exploiting vulnerabilities.
- Manipulating mentees into uncomfortable or unethical situations.
- Showing excessive interest in mentees' personal lives beyond professional boundaries.
- Using mentorship to gain control or exert influence over the mentee's decisions.
- Passing off mentees' work as one's own.

Toxic Leadership
- Frequent displays of anger, condescension, or emotional volatility.
- Setting unrealistic expectations and punishing subordinates for failing to meet them.
- Favoritism or unfairly treating certain team members.
- Discouraging dissent or differing opinions, stifling open communication.
- Blaming others for failures while taking credit for successes.

Dishonesty or Manipulation
- Consistently providing false information or misleading statements.
- Twisting facts to suit personal or organizational agendas.
- Using guilt, fear, or emotional manipulation to control others.
- Making promises that are never fulfilled.
- Withholding crucial information to maintain control.
- Misuse or weaponization of institutional offices, processes and policies.

Unethical Behavior
- Engaging in actions that violate laws or established ethical standards.
- Exploiting vulnerable individuals or groups for personal gain.
- Prioritizing short-term profits or benefits over long-term consequences.
- Engaging in discriminatory practices based on race, gender, or other protected characteristics.

Gaslighting
- Denying the reality of a situation or making someone doubt their own perceptions.
- Manipulating events or conversations to make the victim question their memory.
- Constantly changing the narrative or making inconsistent statements.
- Discrediting the victim's feelings and emotions, making them feel unreasonable.

Notes
_____
_____

References

1. American Medical Association (AMA). What is physician burnout?. Updated February 16, 2023. https://www.ama-assn.org/practice-management/physician-health/what-physician-burnout#:~:text=Physician%20burnout%20is%20an%20epidemic,at%20least%20once%20per%20week. Accessed 4 Mar 2024.
2. Sternberg RJ. Self-sabotage in the academic career. Chronicle of Higher Education. April 29, 2013. https://www.chronicle.com/article/self-sabotage-in-the-academic-career/?sra=true. Accessed 4 Mar 2024.
3. The Chronicle of Higher Education. The dissatisfaction of the associate professor. May 7, 2017. https://www.chronicle.com/article/the-dissatisfaction-of-the-associate-professor/. Accessed 4 Mar 2024.
4. Knight R. How to beat mid-career malaise. Harvard Business Review (HBR). August 2, 2018. https://hbr.org/2018/08/how-to-beat-mid-career-malaise. Accessed 4 Mar 2024.
5. Rosenberg MB. The 4-part nonviolent communication (NVC) process. https://www.nonviolentcommunication.com/learn-nonviolent-communication/4-part-nvc/. Accessed 4 Mar 2024.
6. Rosenberg MB, Chopra D. Nonviolent communication: a language of life: life-changing tools for healthy relationships. PuddleDancer Press; 2015.
7. Kilmann RH. The Thomas-Kilmann Conflict Mode Instrument (TKI). https://kilmanndiagnostics.com/overview-thomas-kilmann-conflict-mode-instrument-tki/. Accessed 4 Mar 2024.
8. American Medical Association (AMA). Why bullying happens in health care and how to stop it. April 2, 2021. https://www.ama-assn.org/practice-management/physician-health/why-bullying-happens-health-care-and-how-stop-it. Accessed 4 Mar 2024.

Further Readings

Harper J. Mobbed: what to do when they are really out to get you. Amazon Books; 2013.
Speak Up Ortho. https://www.speakuportho.org/. Accessed 4 Mar 2024.

Chapter 10
Infusing Diversity into Your Work and Embracing an Inclusive Mindset

As scientists seeking and disseminating truth via systematic inquiry, discovery, treatment, prevention, cure, and education, it's just common sense that science benefits from diverse perspectives. After all, interdisciplinary education and team science have long been celebrated for their ability to break down barriers and drive innovation by bringing together individuals from various backgrounds and disciplines. Yet as my mom used to say, "Common sense isn't so common."

So, what does diversity truly mean on a personal level, beyond its abstract benefits to scientific progress? At its core, diversity is about acknowledging and embracing the unique set of experiences, perspectives, and insights that each person brings to the table; regardless of age, sex, gender identity, race or ethnicity, religion, culture, socioeconomic status, political affiliation, family background, functional ability, etc. It's about understanding that our collective understanding and experience of the world is enriched when we welcome diverse voices and ideas into the conversation [1]. There's a great cartoon (google "cartoon about equity"—credited to Angus Maguire) that nicely illustrates the differences between: *Equality* = when everyone gets the exact same thing; *Equity* = when everyone gets what they need; and *Inclusion/Liberation* = where everyone gets to fully participate. When 'inviting everyone to participate' doesn't seem to be the common practice, you can buck tradition by courageously practicing diversity—not just for the sake of progress, but also for the betterment of your science and the fullness of your life.

And yet, despite this seemingly obvious nature and value of diversity, evidence abounds that we continue to struggle. Why? There's another trite expression our moms used to say: "birds of a feather flock together"; that is, we tend to gravitate towards people who are like us. It's only natural that we feel a sense of comfort and fit with people who *appear* to be similar to us. It's only natural that we may feel some *dis*comfort and *ill*-fit when we're with people who *appear* to be dissimilar to us [2]. The interesting part of this phenomenon is that our brains, in their furious and fast attempts to keep us safe (physically, psychologically, and emotionally), will slap a label on someone as a way of helping us sort-out safety.

Therefore, our challenge is to slow down our thinking (see Daniel Kahneman, Thinking Fast and Slow) and *be more curious and less judgmental* [3]. In the words of Abraham Lincoln, "I do not like that man. I must get to know him better"! When we coach faculty members in difficult situations or mediate conflict, we oftentimes begin with a conversation about what the parties have in common. We ask them to articulate their shared commitment to the work, to fundamental principles and values, to a deep-seated desire to be respected and treated with dignity. That mindset and approach—focusing on commonalities and shared understandings (while being curious and non-judgmental)—will serve you well as you build a purpose-filled career.

You may be thinking or feeling somewhat insulted by the insinuation that you're not already curious and that maybe you're judgmental ("I'm not biased"!). There's a fascinating (and humbling) exercise to test your assumptions called the Harvard Implicit Association Test (Project Implicit). This test is designed to reveal unconscious biases that we may not even be aware of, including those related to gender, race, ethnic groups, religion, skin-tone, sexuality, weight, age, disability, and weapons [4]. We all have prejudices, some of which are deeply ingrained and influence our thoughts and actions without our conscious awareness. The good news is that we can all learn and grow (something scientists love to do). The first step toward growth is awareness.

Self-awareness is the crux of personal development. Recall that "knowing yourself is the beginning of all wisdom" (Aristotle) and "Know Thyself," Socrates). Refer back to Chap. 3 ("Who am I? Why does it matter?") to identify tools that will help you understand your personal preferences, strengths, blind spots, and opportunities for development.

As a faculty member in academic medicine, you have an obligation to yourself, your field, your institution, and the communities you serve. Achieving excellence isn't a solitary endeavor; it thrives within the context of community. Collaboration, diversity, and inclusivity are not just buzzwords; they're the cornerstones of progress and success in any academic pursuit. When you earnestly, purposefully, and humbly dedicate yourself to cultivating diverse and inclusive collaborations, teams, clinics, labs, and beyond, the benefits ripple outward to everyone involved.

The commitment to diversity, equity, and inclusion (DEI) within academic medical centers (AMCs) stems from the recognition that fostering diverse and inclusive environments is both a moral imperative as well as essential for driving innovation and advancing patient care. At institutions like Johns Hopkins Medicine, where DEI is enshrined as a core value, there is a firm acknowledgment of the importance of embracing diverse perspectives and actively promoting equity in healthcare, research, and education.

However, despite these principles being espoused, the reality within academic medicine paints a different picture. The disparities in leadership and faculty representation persist, reflecting the ongoing challenges in translating DEI principles into tangible action and outcomes. For example, even though women comprise nearly half of all medical faculty members, men still greatly outnumber women in dean and department chair roles and at professor rank [5] and faculty members who are Black or African American comprise just 3.9% of full-time faculty at all U.S. medical schools as of 2023, though represent 13.6% of the entire U.S. population [6].

Amidst these disparities, many of our institutions have dedicated offices and appointed leaders who are deeply committed to advancing DEI efforts. The goals of these offices include transforming culture so that all people know and feel that they belong, which is critical to well-being. We are social beings and we all need to feel safe and worthy. Prioritizing belonging enhances the well-being and success of our faculty, staff, and learners, while also strengthening our academic communities, driving innovation and excellence.

However, higher education is currently facing backlash regarding its DEI efforts. This trend reflects a broader resistance to acknowledging and addressing systemic inequity in our society, as well as a reluctance to confront uncomfortable truths about the barriers faced by marginalized groups. Some institutions have responded to pressure or legislation by renaming offices or rebranding initiatives, while continuing to carry out the essential work of advancing DEI. However, simply changing the name of a DEI office does not erase the importance or need for its work. And it does not ameliorate the investment we all share in the well-being of our colleagues and learners. Nothing prohibits us as individuals from adopting an inclusive mindset and taking deliberate steps to foster belonging. If you, or any of your colleagues or learners experience discriminatory behavior, microaggressions/microinequities, a hostile work environment, or unjust 'minority taxes,' related to any aspect of your identity (e.g., race, ethnicity, background, gender identity, religion, age, weight, politics, ability, etc.), these offices and leaders are there for support.

We can all do better to be more open, more curious, and less judgmental. Embracing an inclusive mindset and practice will enable us to recruit, retain, promote, and build the best faculty and leadership teams to educate learners and serve our patients and communities. It's just good, common sense.

Points to Ponder
- What are my implicit biases? How do they affect who I include, how I treat patients, or otherwise approach my work?
- How can I leverage my advantages and disadvantages to help others?
- What do diversity and inclusivity look like in my spheres? What voices are missing from my team(s)?
- Who amongst my closest colleagues/friends do I trust to tell me the truth about my areas for growth?
- How can I challenge myself to get more comfortable in my discomfort?

Notes

References

1. Servaes S, Choudhury P, Parikh AK. What is diversity? Pediatr Radiol. 2022;52(9):1708–10.
2. Verkuyten M, Yogeeswaran K. Cultural diversity and its implications for intergroup relations. Curr Opin Psychol. 2020;(32):1–5. https://doi.org/10.1016/j.copsyc.2019.06.010. Accessed 5 Mar 2024.
3. Kahneman D. Thinking, fast and slow. New York: Farrar, Straus, and Giroux; 2011.
4. Harvard Implicit Association Test. Project Implicit. https://implicit.harvard.edu/implicit/takeatest.html. Accessed 5 Mar 2024.
5. AAMC Faculty Roster. 2023 U.S. Medical School Faculty. 2023 Report. Table 3. https://www.aamc.org/media/8481/download?attachment. Accessed 5 Mar 2024.
6. United States Census Bureau. Quick Facts. United States. https://www.census.gov/quickfacts/fact/table/US/RHI225222 Accessed 5 Mar 2024.

Chapter 11
The Work-Life Integration Paradox

Work doesn't love you back. This doesn't mean that you shouldn't love your job. Hopefully, you do, or you will by following the guidance in this book. After all, you made a lot of sacrifices to get to where you are; not to mention that directly impacting people's lives and the scientific field is inherently meaningful and purposeful. It's often for these very reasons that faculty in academic medicine have a propensity to overwork [1].

Which is why this chapter is not a traditional interpretation of work-life integration, in the sense of how you can juggle a demanding career, caretaking responsibilities, hobbies, and even take a guilt-free vacation once in a while. There is enough out there on that topic. I'm willing to bet that you've already read things and listened to podcasts about it. You've likely adopted some hacks, like the Pomodoro technique or a color-coded calendar. And you still have too much work and not enough time. That's why this chapter endeavors to help you gain a broader perspective on the role of work in the context of your life, with the objective of you determining for yourself what is most important and to allocate your time accordingly.

Chances are pretty good that if you're reading this book, you are a high-achiever. This stems in part from our society, which is achievement-oriented. Many of us want, or say we want, a balanced life, one that harmoniously makes room for both work and everything else in our lives. Though in reality, many of us allow work to occupy a large portion of the space allocated to "everything else."

This is in part because work is designed to reward achievement-oriented people. Consider your institution's measures of success, the factors cited in your annual review—number of papers published, classes taught, trainees mentored, patient volume, grant dollars brought in, etc. These are all ways in which productivity is measured, although the validity of these measures as true indicators of performance are suspect. Nonetheless, institutions know that achievement-oriented people love to meet and exceed an expectation, so they incentivize us to keep working by measuring things that require a good amount of our time. These are known as "carrots."

Then there are "sticks." Sticks are forms of punishment for not achieving certain types of metrics. Sticks are commonly applied when the activity is not that inherently rewarding, such as closing notes or doing safety training. Many institutions have implemented policies that deduct vacation days, bonus potential, or at the very least publicly shame employees who don't complete the assigned activity within a certain amount of time.

Both of these mechanisms activate the achievement mindset. And both mechanisms contribute to overwork. Meanwhile, what is happening in our personal lives? In terms of our relationships or hobbies, nothing is being measured. Not in the way that activates the achievement mindset anyway. Though we might set some goals for ourselves such as wanting to get married, have children, buy our first house, or play tennis a couple times a week, those types of life goals aren't as tangible or time-bound as work goals. And let's say we are partnered, have kids, own a house and play tennis a couple times a week, does this mean we have it all and therefore have found balance? Unlikely.

The most likely scenario is that no matter what, we feel constantly overwhelmed. We take on task after task, fueling the achievement-mindset, causing us to remain rooted in doing too much in all facets of life in an attempt to get the dopamine hits that come from achievement. And then, at some point, life happens in a way that can't be ignored. For many of us, that was the pandemic. It could also be the need to care for aging parents, the death of a close loved one, or a significant illness. For many people, women in particular, it's the birth of a child. These events present stark contrasts to the achievement-orientation of professional life.

In these moments, the conventional measures of success and achievement lose their luster. Questions arise about the meaning of life and what really matters. We then fully experience love, gratitude, and are able to let the little things slide. Through this lens, we begin to view work for what it is, a means to express our talent and potential and contribute to the world, not our sole reason for being. In these times we learn life lessons. But often, we revert back to work because there we feel productive, our progress is measurable, our contributions vital.

How can we get the same type of reward from all facets of our lives? The trick of the work-life integration paradox is to define success and fulfillment on our terms. In essence, to see the forest for the trees. To make a real shift in your mindset, start by evaluating your day-to-day experiences. Are you feeling fulfilled and satisfied, or are you pushing yourself to the point of burnout? Consider the satisfaction you get from your achievements. Do they truly make you happy, or are you just ticking off boxes to meet others' expectations? Think about why you do what you do. Are you striving for personal fulfillment or chasing after external approval? [2] Know that you are enough—right now, as you are—and that you don't need anyone else's approval. Are you comparing yourself to others? Know that comparison is the thief of joy.

If so, go back to Chap. 3 (Who am I? Why does it matter?) where we urged you to explore your values and who you are. Now, revisit your values in the context of time. Are you allocating your time in a way that aligns with your values and brings genuine satisfaction? Consider if you are keeping yourself busy to attempt to avoid the discomfort not being fulfilled? Embrace the idea that success doesn't always adhere to a predefined timeline and that the path to fulfillment may involve detours and unexpected turns.

Practicing mindfulness can be a powerful tool in this process. By being present in the moment, you can appreciate the richness of everyday experiences, whether at work or in your personal life. Mindfulness allows you to savor the journey rather than fixate solely on the destination, fostering a sense of contentment irrespective of external markers of success [3].

Cultivating a supportive community can also be instrumental in navigating this paradigm shift. Surround yourself with individuals who share similar values and understand the importance of a holistic approach to life. Engage in open conversations about redefining success, exchanging insights, and supporting each other's journeys.

The work-life integration paradox challenges you to question societal norms and typical success measures. Make deliberate choices that align with what genuinely matters to you. This isn't about being complacent; it's about consciously shaping your life in a way that integrates all aspects. It's easy to get caught up in the hustle and responding to others' needs. True fulfillment comes from expressing your talents in a way that serves both you and the world.

Now, consider the long term. Picture your retirement, a stage of life often romanticized as a time of relaxation and fulfillment. How do you want to look back on your career and life journey at that point? What kind of legacy do you want to leave? How do you want to be remembered? The choices you make today shape not only your present but also your future. By aligning your choices with your values and finding harmony between work and personal life, you're not just preparing for retirement; you're actively creating a future that reflects the richness of a life lived to the fullest.

The work-life integration paradox is not a puzzle to be solved definitively; rather, it's an ongoing exploration of what it means to live a fulfilling life. Challenging conventional measures of success, reassessing values, and embracing intentional choices *is* integration. Or, as is often said, no one lays on their death bed wishing they had worked more.

Points to Ponder
- What sticks and carrots dictate the way I spend my time?
- How do I define meaning in my life?
- How can I devote less time to others' sticks and carrots and more time to what is personally meaningful to me?
- If I pretend I'm 70 and looking back at my life, what advice can I give my present self?
- How and where would my life benefit from mindfulness?

Notes

_____
_____
_____

References

1. Shanafelt TD, Hasan O, Dyrbye LN, Sinsky C, Satele D, Sloan J, West CP. Changes in burnout and satisfaction with work-life balance in physicians and the general US working population between 2011 and 2014. Mayo Clin Proc. 2015;90(12):1600–13.
2. Wei JL, Villwock JA. Balance versus integration: work-life considerations. Otolaryngol Clin N Am. 2021;54(4):823–37.
3. Karakash S, Solone M, Chavez J, Shanafelt T. Physician work-life integration: challenges and strategies for improvement. Clin Obstet Gynecol. 2019;62(3):455–65.

Further Reading

McKeown G. Essentialism: this disciplined pursuit of less currency. New York: Currency, Crown Publishing Group; 2014.

Chapter 12
Transitions

In academic medicine, career stages are typically characterized as early-career, mid-career, and later-career. There are no age delineations or qualifiers for these stages; rather, they're latent constructs for broadly characterizing the faculty life cycle in academia. Early-career is when we just start-out, usually at the assistant professor rank. Mid-career is typically when we've reached associate professor status and have 'gotten the hang of it.' Later-career is approximately 7–10+ years after associate professor, sometimes with designations such as tenure or full professor status. Recently, many academic institutions have been paying more attention to the mid- and later-career faculty members than in the past because the mean age for faculty members is increasing. According to the most recent AAMC Faculty Roster data (December 31, 2023), 43% of full-time medical school faculty are age 50+ and the average age of medical school faculty in 2023 was 49.2 years [1].

Coupled with the projected shortages of physicians, institutions are starting to pay greater attention to the wants and needs of their later-career faculty members. For example, in later life, many people are providing care for aging parents, extended family members, and spouses or partners [2]. Our (Kim) recent paper found that 19% of full-time faculty members age 55+ reported providing care on an on-going basis to a family member, friend, or neighbor with a chronic illness or disability, of which 90% reported experiencing some or a lot of mental or emotional strain from caregiving [3].

If you are in the later-career phase or in a leadership role, learn about the programs and resources that are available to later-career faculty members. These include a wide array of traditional resources through your human resources offices, such as health care benefits, disability, FMLA, retirement planning, etc. Additionally, faculty development offices may offer seminars, workshops, or retreats to develop strategies for life after full-time employment. Transitioning to retirement is often challenging for faculty in academic medicine because their identity is so tied to their career [4, 5]. Therefore, exploring questions such as: who am I after I leave academic medicine? what will I do? what will my purpose be? and how will I build new networks and communities? can help smooth your transition. In addition, your institution may have a 'retirement academy' or similar organization where can build community with other academics who are also exploring part-time employment, consulting, mentoring and coaching, traveling, volunteering, etc. Your "next chapter" after full-time work may not be retirement as much as it may be replenishment. You may have opportunity to do the things you've always wanted to do, like: write a book; read books for fun; spend more time with family; travel; volunteer; learn something new; train for a marathon; learn to play pickleball, or discover something else that delights you.

Although retirement is a significant transition, you'll have many transition points throughout your career. We all experience gains and losses; which can be positive or negative. *Positive gains* include: educational degrees; licenses; credentials; jobs; ranks; titles/roles; partners; children and family; hobbies; and friends. *Negative gains* include just about everything in the prior sentence! As curious academics who value education and constantly seek more knowledge, we tend to collect projects like pet rocks. These pet rock projects result in increased responsibilities which make for hard decisions when it comes time to start thinking about what we're going to give up. Our personal gains and joys inevitably result in competing demands on our time.

Just like positive gains can be both good and bad, losses can also be both good and bad. *Negative losses* will include: departing loved ones; short-term and long-term health challenges; and many job-related losses such as decreased or discontinued grant funding, manuscript rejections, unscored grant applications, faculty/staff turnover, changes in institutional leadership, etc. Some of those losses will be good for us. *Positive losses* include those silver-lining moments that may not be realized until after the effect. For example, that rejected manuscript will be revised and accepted somewhere else. That grant application will get better and get funded. That bad leader will move on and that job you didn't get will open the door for an even better opportunity. An important point is to remind yourself that life will happen, regardless of your planning—or not planning. Focus on that which you can control—you and your behavioral responses!

As your career progresses, you will be offered many opportunities. As you grow in your professional arena, develop your niche expertise, become nationally and internationally known, take-on leadership roles in your professional societies, institutions, and communities, you will be sought-out to share your wisdom. Be prudent (i.e., judicious, practical, sensible, wise, careful, cautious). As opportunities arise, take your time to reflect on your values, purpose, mission, and goals. If you don't know—and periodically reflect on—your: values and beliefs, purpose, mission, and goals, you may find yourself disconnected from your *self* (once again, refer to Chap. 3—we seem to send you back to that chapter more than any other). After careful introspection about new internal or external opportunities, convene your inner circle of mentors and lean on their wisdom and experience to help you gauge your decisions.

There are myriad leadership opportunities in academic medicine. However, before you start thinking about positional leadership roles, such as program, division, and department directors, chiefs, CEOs, deans, provosts and the like, know what you will be giving up to take one on. Many view a leadership role as the next step in a career trajectory, not being fully aware of the requirement *to lead*. This means to be in service to others, and that often comes at the expense of your own ambitions. One of the key reasons that leaders in academic medicine fail is because they remain too committed to *their* research programs, *their* clinical practice, *their* publication record, and ignore *their* responsibility to grow and develop others. Therefore, per our usual advice, take some time and space and seek wise counsel before you accept additional roles and responsibilities.

Similarly, other institutions and/or industries will seek expertise and try to recruit you. The same advice applies here. The grass may look greener elsewhere, but you must know that no place is perfect and that every institution has its challenges. Know the difference between when you 'just need a break' and when you need to 'break free.'

You may just need a break when you are experiencing burnout, which is endemic in academic medicine (see Chap. 9: "What to do when (not if) things get rough"). You will undoubtedly have seasons and moments in your career where you are feeling burned out. You will not be alone; your colleagues and team members are or have been burned out as well [6]. In addition to investing in self-care via adequate sleep, nutrition, breathing, exercise, socializing, and whatever else you need to nourish your brain, body, heart, and soul, you may consider taking a break via a vacation or a sabbatical. It's been my (Kim) experience that academic medicine faculty members don't take enough vacation time; and when they do, they still do work! Paradoxically, taking vacation results in us being more productive [7]. Try a real vacation, disconnected from email and work texts.

In addition, your institution may provide sabbaticals, which we've noticed is something that academic medicine faculty members rarely take [8]. Sabbatical leaves are designed to provide rest and recovery from usual work duties. Traditionally, faculty members on sabbatical engage in self-directed study or research elsewhere [9]. Explore your institution's policies and departmental precedents for sabbaticals and do some research on what your colleagues have done. I (Kim) recently heard one of our department directors say that he has given his faculty mini, 2-week sabbaticals to finish writing a paper or a grant application! Who knew? You won't know—unless you ask! If sabbaticals are not offered or you are not eligible, consider creating your own! We are so conditioned to believe that we have to keep working no matter what, that unless something tragic happens that requires us to take a break, we don't. There are other types of leave available, including unpaid leave. Should you choose to take a break, you might take some time to write, learn a new technique or skill, do an intern-/externship somewhere, be a visiting scholar, get a master's degree, travel, serve...the possibilities are as vast as your imagination.

If you think you need to break free, in addition to some serious personal reflection and seeking the counsel of wise colleagues, friends, and family members, you may want to invest in a professional career coach. We coach many faculty members who are being recruited or who are looking for new frontiers elsewhere. A coach will help you clarify your values, goals, obstacles, options, and action steps. A coach will also help you negotiate the offer (because you should *always* negotiate).

One important warning here—don't ever use a real or possible job offer as a threat at your current institution. It's an unfortunate reality that many institutions will not offer a retention package without another offer in hand or won't even give you a counter-offer! There's also no guarantee that even if your current institution does provide you with a counter-offer it will even suit your needs. So if you pursue this route, you must be prepared to leave. That is, you should not engage in 'the job market' if you have no real intentions of moving institutions; you're wasting others' and your own time and possibly building a bad reputation among recruiters and other institutions if you start going on interviews merely to game the system. If you do decide to move, do so with professionalism and grace and don't speak badly about past institutions or people; you never know when opportunities may arise and you find yourself full-circle back from whence you came or 'that person you trash-talked' comes to your new institution!

You may also be curious about careers and life outside of academic medicine. It's not uncommon for clinicians, investigators, and health care professionals to move to industry; and even though it is often said that once you move out of academia, you can't come back, but this is not true. There are always roles and pathways back; they just may not always be obvious. You can certainly learn more about private practice, pharma, government, business, tech firms, etc. from colleagues, your professional societies, your institution's innovation or tech start-up centers, and via social media platforms such as LinkedIn. Explore, innovate, incorporate your entrepreneurial curiosity into your current academic portfolio! If you become serious about moving to industry, working with a recruiting firm and/or a coach will help you identify transferable skills and translate your accomplishments to corporate-speak.

Much like the guidance given throughout this entire book, there is no one right way or time to make a transition. Transition points in one's career can be daunting, yet they also offer opportunities for growth and renewal. Whether it's advancing through promotional ranks, embracing leadership roles, or overcoming hurdles and challenges, each transition presents a chance to reassess goals, refine strategies, and pursue new avenues of development. It's not just about reaching a destination but embracing the journey, armed with knowledge, self-awareness, and a commitment to continuous growth.

As you venture forth on your academic journey, remember that you're not alone. This book stands as a companion, offering guidance, support, and practical advice to help you navigate the twists and turns of your career path. Our hope is that you'll emerge from these pages with a clearer sense of direction, a deeper understanding of yourself, and the tools you need to thrive in the ever-evolving landscape of academic medicine. It's essential to reflect on the central message of this book: that focusing on your overarching career and professional development is the key to having a fulfilling, aligned, and successful career in academic medicine. Inner knowing is the most valuable gift you can give yourself.

Points to Ponder
- Do I use all or most of my vacation time each year? If not, why not? When I take vacation, do I work, am I rejuvenated? How can I build-in time to restore?

- Who is in my inner circle of advisors?
- What are my thoughts about retirement? What might be written in my "next chapter?"
- How do I know if I need a break or need to break free?
- How can I explore my opportunities? What's my plan?

Notes

_____
_____
_____

References

1. AAMC Faculty Roster: 2023 U.S. Medical School Faculty. 2023 Report. Appendix Tables G & H. https://www.aamc.org/media/8481/download?attachment. Accessed 5 Mar 2024.
2. Levine RB, Walling A, Chatterjee A, Skarupski KA. Factors influencing retirement decisions of senior faculty at US medical schools: are there gender-based differences? J Women's Health. 2022;31(7):974–82.
3. Skarupski KA, Roth DL, Durso SC. Prevalence of caregiving and high caregiving strain among late-career medical school faculty members: workforce, policy, and faculty development implications. Hum Resour Health. 2021;19(36):1–9. https://doi.org/10.1186/s12960-021-00582-3.
4. Skarupski KA. Invited chapter. Managing Career transitions and succession. AAMC GFA Guidebook. Co-editors: Gibson J, Freeman E, Ripley B, Hill J, Brazeau C, Rowland M, Best B, Love J, Runge C. September 2020. https://www.aamc.org/professional-development/affinity-groups/gfa/leadership-guide-faculty-affairs-professionals.
5. Skarupski KA. Invited chapter. In: Busby-Whitehead J, Durso S, Arenson C, Palmer M, Elon R, Reichel W, editors. Reichel's care of the elderly, 8th ed. Chapter 57. Retirement: a contemporary perspective. Cambridge: Cambridge University Press; 2021.
6. West CP, Dyrbye LN, Shanafelt TD. Physician burnout: contributors, consequences, and solutions. J Intern Med. 2018;283(6):516–29.
7. Zucke R.. How taking a vacation improves your well-being. Harvard Business Review. July 19, 2023. https://hbr.org/2023/07/how-taking-a-vacation-improves-your-well-being. Accessed 5 Mar 2024.
8. Robiner WN, Thompson Buum H, Eckerstorfer M, Kim MH, Kirsch JD. Sabbaticals in US medical schools. Am J Med. 2023;136(3):322–8. https://doi.org/10.1016/j.amjmed.2022.11.007.
9. Gardner SK. Faculty learning and professional growth in the sabbatical leave. Innov High Educ. 2022;47(3):435–51.

Further Readings

Skarupski KA, Welch C, Dandar V, Mylona E, Chatterjee A, Singh M. Late-career expectations: a survey of full-time faculty members who are 55 or older at 14 U.S. medical schools. Acad Med. 2020;95(2):226–33.

Skarupski KA, Dandar V, Mylona E, Chatterjee A, Welch C, Singh M. Late career faculty: a survey of faculty affairs and faculty development leaders of U.S. medical schools. Acad Med. 2020;95(2):234–40.

Index

A
Abusive behaviors, 53, 54
Academic freedom, 7, 8
Academic health centers (AHCs), 1
   aims, 2
   being recruited, 67
   school of medicine, 1
Academic medicine
   academic freedom, 7, 8
   career stages, early career/mid-career/late-career, 65
   clinical trials, observational studies/basic science research, 8
   diversity, 58
   faculty, 3
   faculty members, 2
   faculty rank and promotion, 9, 10
   healthcare policy researchers, 8
   medical educators, 8
   mission, 1, 28
      aims, 2
      community engagement, 2
      faculty members, 2, 3
      innovation, 2
      patient care, 2
      research, 2
      salaries, 4
      service, 1
      teaching, 2
   overview, 1
   patient care, 1
   patient outcomes, 9
   researching job opportunities (*see* Researching job opportunities)
   scholarship, 7
   teaching, 7
Appointments, promotion and tenure document, 29

B
Boyer's classification of scholarship, 7, 39
Burnout, 3, 12, 29, 41, 42, 49
   aspirations, 29
   coping with, 49
   overwork, 29
   self-care, 67

C
Career, 3
   fulfillment, 11
   progression, 33
   scholarship, 28
Career setbacks
   assessing risk, 52
   bullying, 51
   burnout, 49
   career coach, seeking help, 51
   challenges, 49, 50
   dysfunction and toxicity, 52
   harassment, 51
   harassment, how to address, 51
      escalation, 52
   HR and management, 51–52
   institution's Office of Institutional Equity (OIE), 52
   learning from, 50
   legal guidance, 52
   mid-career, 51

Career setbacks (cont.)
    procrastination, perfectionism, imposter syndrome, 50
    self-awareness, 50
    self-sabotage, 50
    stress, 50
    support with, 53
    university reputation/personal safety, 52
Career stages
    associate professor, 41
    boundaries, 41
    care-giving, 65
    early career, 9
    full professor, 41
    late-career, 9
    mid-career, 9
CliftonStrengths, 13
Coaching, 15
Community hospital, 1
Continuing education unit (CEUs), 34
Continuing medical education (CME), 34
Culture, 20, 26
    promotion and, 39

D
Diversity
    communities, 58
    experiences, perspectives, and insights, 57
    healthcare, research, and education, 58
    innovation and excellence, 59
    judgmental thinking, 58
    leadership and faculty representation, 58, 59
    non-judgmental thinking, 58
    resources and support, 59
    self-awareness, 58
    systemic inequity, 59
Diversity, equity, and inclusion, 43

E
Eisenhower Matrix, 32
Emotional intelligence (EI), 13, 44
Enneagram, 13

F
Faculty, 2
    allied health professionals, 1, 3
    appointment terms, 28
    contracts, 3
    job security, 3
    leadership roles, 3
    niche, reputation, 29
    physician, 3
    position type, protected time, 20
    professional development programs, 34
    ranks, 9
    role, 3
        basic scientists, 8
        clinician-scientists, 8
        healthcare policy researchers, 8
        medical educators, 8
        scholar, 8
        triple threat, 2–3
    salary, 3
    salary ranges, 4
    scientist, 3
    tenure, 3
    track and path, 19
        adjunct, 19
        auxiliary, 19
        clinical track, 19
        clinician-educator, 19
        practice track, 19
        "regular" faculty, 19
        research track, 19
        tenure track, 19, 40
    types of scholars, 8
Faculty development
    See also Professional development

G
Gallup, 13
Grant funding, obtaining, 34

I
Impact, 8, 39
    demonstration of, 9
    disseminating outcomes, 28
    patient outcomes, 8
Inclusion
    belonging, 25, 43, 59 (*see also* Diversity)
    implicit bias, 58
Influence, 26
    positional authority, 26
    relational authority, 26
Interview, 18
Invited presentation, 46
    how to get, 46

Index

J
Job search
  coaching services, 18
  contract review, 21
  counter-offer, 68
  culture, 20
  curriculum vitae (C.V.), 18
  how to evaluate, 20
  interview, 20
  interview preparation, 18
  leadership role, 46
  negotiation, 20, 21
    salary/compensation, 20
  offer letter, 21
  on-campus visit, 19
  on-campus visit, preparing for, 18
  retention package, 68
  social media platforms, 68
  values, 21

L
Leadership, 47
  annual review, 46
  behaviors, 43
  career stages, early-career, 44, 46
  competencies (*see also* Professional development)
  conferences, 45
  emotional intelligence, 47
  followership, 46, 47
  getting noticed, 46
  group dynamics, 44
  interpersonal relationships, 44
  job sites, 46
  networking, 46
  nominations, 45
  organizational impact, 43, 44
  overview, 43
  positional leadership, 43
  positions, applying for, 46
  professional society, 45
  programs, 45 (*see also* Professional Development)
  reputation, 46
  resources, 45
  roles, 44
  self-awareness, 43, 44
  skills, 43, 44
  team leadership, 44
  training (*see also* Professional development)
Leadership development
  career stages, 45 (*see also* professional development)
Leadership position, how to get, 46

M
Menteeship, how to, 26
Mentorship, 7, 9
  how to find, 25
  peer mentorship, 25
  research, 33
Mentors, types of, 25, 26
Myers-Briggs Type Indicator (MBTI), 13

N
National Institutes of Health (NIH), 34
Negotiation
  non-negotiables, 21
  offer letter, 28
  salary, 20
Networking, 23, 34
  administrative staff, 25
  authority, 26
  barriers, 27, 28
  conferences, 33
  decision-making, 27
  email, 24, 25
  faculty development, 25
  goal, 23
  how to, 24
  influence, 27
  information and connection, 25
  mentors, 26
  mindset, 23
  objectives, 24
  onboarding plan, 24
  opportunities and recommendations, 25
  organizational focus, 27
  politics, 26, 27
  problem-solving, 26, 27
  relationship-building, 26
  scholarship, 28, 29
Niche, 28
  how to, 28

O
Office politics, 26
  how to navigate, 27
Onboarding, 24, 28, 31
  how to, 25
  types of, 33
Organizational "org" charts, 24

P

Peer-review, how to, 33
Positional authority, 26
Positional leadership, 43
Professional career development plan
    (PCDP), 44
Professional development, 2, 34
    boundary setting, 33
    career development, 9
    continuing medical education (CME)/
        continuing education units
        (CEU), 34
    5-year plan, 29
    life satisfaction, 12
    mission statements, 14
    Office of Faculty Development, 34
    self-assessment tools, 12
        CliftonStrengths, 12
        EI assessment, 13
        Enneagram, 13
        Myers-Briggs Type Indicator
            (MBTI), 13
        360 Assessment, 13
        VIA Character Assessment, 13
    self-awareness, 15
    vision statement, 14
Professional identity
    expertise, 28
    mission statements, 15
    niche, 28
    process of, 11
    purpose, 14
    retirement, 65
    satisfaction in life, 12
    self-awareness, 11, 12, 15
    sense of fulfillment, 12
    values, 12, 13
    values, purpose, mission, and goals, 66
    vision statement, 14
Promotion
    annual review, 40
    appointments, promotion and tenure
        document, 38
    to associate professor, 41
    associate professor, what to expect, 41
    committees and service activities, 41
    credibility, 40
    criteria, 9, 38
    demystifying, 37
    denial, 39
    dossier, 29, 39, 46
    excellence and reputation, 38
    external review, 39
    extramural funding, 38
    faculty member, 37
    to full professor, 41
    full professor, how to, 41
    how to get promoted, 38
    impact, 9
    information, 39
    invited presentation, 46
    and leadership, 37, 41
    metrics, 38
    niche, 42
    office politics, 38
    overview, 37
    peer-review, 39
    priorities and goals, 41
    professional credibility, 40
    reputation, 9, 38, 41
    reputation building, 39, 40
    rules and guidelines, 37
    scholarship, 39
    shifting priorities, 38
    talents, skills, and interests, 37
    time frame/"clock", 40
    track and path, 37, 38
        rank, 9
    values, mission and vision, 41

R

Relational authority, 26
Reputation
    establishing, 23
    how to build, 27
    niche, 28
Reputation building
    being recommended, 40
    how to, 40
Research, 7
    types of research, 8
Researching job opportunities
    AAMC CareerConnect, 18
    The Chronicle of Higher Education jobs
        site, 18
    clinical practice/teaching, 17
    HigherEdJobs, 18
    job application, 18
    mission, vision, and values statements, 18
    negotiating job offers, 21
    on-campus visit, 19
    position type, 17, 18
    qualities, 18
Research program
    funding opportunities, 34
    how to build, 33

Index

S
Scholarship, 7
  accountability, 32
  career progress, 33
  CEUs, 34
  CME, 34
  conferences, 33
  faculty members, 34
  funded grant applications, 34
  NIH, 34
  overview, 31
  patient and clinic responsibilities, 32
  peer review, 33
  research program, 34
  setting boundaries, 32, 33
  time management, 32
  types of scholars
    basic scientists, 8
    clinician-scientists, 8
    health policy researchers, 8
    medical educators, 8
  WAG, 31, 32
  writing, 32

T
Teaching, 7, 8
  educator, 29
Tenure, 3, 9
Time management, 32
  Eisenhower Matrix, 33
  teaching and scholarship prioritization, 33
Transitions, 68
  burnout, 67
  career progression, 66
  fulfillment, 68
  gains and losses, 66
  knowledge, self-awareness, and commitment, 68
  move to industry, 68
  opportunities, 66, 67
  positional leadership, 66
  priorities and goals, professional career coach, 23
  professional career coach, 67
  promotion, 68
  resources, 65
  retention package, 68
  retirement, 65, 66
  sabbatical, 67
  shortages of physicians, 65
  transition points, 66

V
Values, 11, 23, 43, 46

W
Work-life integration
  achievement mindset, 62
  achievement-orientation, 61
  annual review, 61
  community, 63
  fulfillment, 63
  metrics, 62
  mindfulness, 63
  mindset shift, 62
  overwork, 61
  paradox, 61
  success and fulfillment, 62, 63
  time management, 61
  values, 62
  what really matters, 62
Writing accountability group (WAG), 31, 32, 44
  how to set up, 32

GPSR Compliance

The European Union's (EU) General Product Safety Regulation (GPSR) is a set of rules that requires consumer products to be safe and our obligations to ensure this.

If you have any concerns about our products, you can contact us on ProductSafety@springernature.com

In case Publisher is established outside the EU, the EU authorized representative is:

Springer Nature Customer Service Center GmbH
Europaplatz 3
69115 Heidelberg, Germany

Batch number: 09745535

Printed by Printforce, the Netherlands